THE ROLE OF CITRUS
IN HEALTH AND DISEASE

THE ROLE OF CITRUS
IN HEALTH AND DISEASE

Willard A. Krehl

A University of Florida Book

The University Presses of Florida
Gainesville / 1976

Library of Congress Cataloging in Publication Data

Krehl, Willard A
 The role of citrus in health and disease.

 "A University of Florida book."
 Bibliography: p.
 1. Nutrition. 2. Citrus fruits. 3. Vitamin C.
I. Title.
RA784.K73   613.2'6   76–4502
ISBN 0-8130-0532-9
ISBN 0-8130-0571-X   pbk.

PRINTED BY ROSE PRINTING COMPANY, TALLAHASSEE, FLORIDA

Contents

Foreword

This volume is unique in that it deals with a commodity or group of foods, and, at the same time, presents a broad coverage of scientific information about nutrition and its role in the prevention of disease and the maintenance of health. The major goal is to present important findings relating nutrition to health; in fact, it is clearly recognized that food and nutrition are key components in the prevention of disease. The author delineates the nutritional value of citrus, particularly orange juice, and identifies the continuing role played by the Florida Citrus Commission in insuring product quality for the consumer. The function of essential nutrients, especially those provided by citrus products, is discussed in considerable detail.

In an era of health care in which greater emphasis is placed on the prevention of disease through earlier identification of risk factors and their reduction in the individual, the nutritional approach in the preventive process makes a great deal of common sense. This book therefore should be useful and of interest to a wide spectrum of members of the health care team including physicians, dentists, nurses, and dietitians. The style of presentation and content should also make interesting reading for the intelligent and interested layman.

Through summary and evaluation an appreciation of sound nutritional concepts and their application in both preventive and therapeutic medicine are presented.

GRACE GOLDSMITH, M.D.
Professor of Nutrition
Tulane University

General Introduction

Two earlier editions of *Citrus Fruits in Health and Disease* prepared for the medical and health professions and published in 1948 and 1956, respectively, presented critical and then current reviews of the pertinent scientific and clinical literature identifying the appropriate place of citrus products and their major nutrients, particularly ascorbic acid, in the maintenance of health and in the prevention of disease (1, 2). Each of these editions provided basic information on the composition of citrus products, including the then most recent analytical data available, particularly with respect to essential nutrient composition. The role of citrus fruits and their important nutrients in the management of disease, as published in the clinical literature, has traditionally been reviewed with an eye toward critical evaluation. This book continues to identify the role of citrus and its nutrients in the normal nutritional process and in the management of disease, but it is quite evident that a new perspective is at hand and deserving of emphasis. *This new perspective is an emphasis on disease prevention and on the maintenance of health through the use of a more appropriate selection of foods and nutrients (3–7).* In part, this is a reflection of the changing emphasis in medicine itself. The clinical practice of medicine has become an increasingly sophisticated science with a concentration on targeted therapy, particularly with specific drugs directed to specific points in the metabolic pathways at the molecular and enzymatic levels of the cell. The broad spectrum of nutrients in a food such as citrus is not easily applicable to the targeted therapy concept commonly employed in the controlled clinical study or in the clinical research center. This

1

is not to imply that a food, such as citrus, does not have a continuing importance in the maintenance of health and in the overall medical therapeutic regimen directed at sick people, but it is difficult and yet necessary to identify the precise role that a particular nutrient exerts at the enzymatic and molecular levels within the cell in a controlled study with a minimum of variables. In this context, food, any food, represents primarily a substantial number of chemical substances or nutrients which mix into the total pool of absorbed nutrients and are utilized and metabolized at the cellular level to maintain health or augment therapy in the treatment of disease. More important, each nutrient or chemical in this metabolic mix may exert a separate and isolated effect, or the therapeutic effect measured may be mediated by an entirely unappreciated interaction of the "mix" of nutrients or by the "imbalance" of the nutrients created in the metabolic pool (8). Citrus is above all a food and is usually ingested in its near natural state which is not significantly altered by processing. It certainly contains an excellent blend of nutrients known to be important for health and significant in the treatment and management of a number of diseases. Medical claims reported in the scientific literature for any of the nutrients in citrus, or in any food, are often based on isolated studies with a specific nutrient, under circumstances not necessarily characteristic of a food containing that nutrient. Studies using huge doses of ascorbic acid represent a prime example of this; the results obtained are not to be interpreted as an effect of citrus. Therefore, one who critically evaluates the claims regarding the effects of citrus, or any food with a mix of nutrients, must recognize the difficulty of attributing specific or special merits or faults to the food as it relates to any single nutrient.

Another new concept is that nutrients may have a physiological or pharmacologic utility over and above their usual nutritional function. Thus, we entertain the idea of "orthomolecular medicine" with certain implied therapeutic or preventive claims for certain nutrients at dose levels that far exceed any recognized nutritional concept that has been ascribed to the nutrient in question, i.e., ascorbic acid (vitamin C) (9). There is little doubt, therefore, that we are embarking on a new era of experimentation and clinical application utilizing nutrients at "megadose" levels far in excess of their traditional requirements. It is also clear that this new concept has produced substantial controversy between the "traditional" nutritional point of view and the "megavitamin" theory. This new perspective must then be reviewed and discussed with the concept of targeted "meganutrient" therapy at the cellular or molecular level as the main focus.

Regardless of the controversy of "normal" nutrient levels versus "megavitamin" therapy, citrus fruits remain important and practical daily dietary sources of ascorbic acid as well as other nutrients necessary for the maintenance of health and in the management of disease. We should not lose sight of the simple fact that fresh citrus fruits or processed citrus products and juices (particularly orange juice) represent practical, palatable, readily available, and inexpensive sources not only of vitamin C but of other key nutrients as well. Again the accent is on citrus as a food, not as a medication.

A major premise in this review is that the prevention of disease will, in fact, be the next "great wave" in medicine even though the concepts of disease prevention and nutritional science are as old as Hippocrates, who advocated nutrition first, then drugs, then surgery. Prevention, by every means available, is essential if we are to make a significant impact on the major chronic and debilitating diseases, such as coronary heart disease, cancer, and stroke. Our current medical care system with its emphasis on crisis medical problems has had only a very modest effect in reducing morbidity and mortality from these diseases. Although slightly more than 10 per cent of the American population is over 65 years of age, and this percentage is increasing continuously, life expectancy, particularly for the American male, has not increased significantly in the last twenty-five years. This means that increasingly we are succumbing prematurely to those diseases that are major causes of mortality. Some say that this is a result of the stress imposed by our society, and no doubt this is a factor, as well as are the personality characteristics and the life style of many individuals. The continued development of nutritional science and the sound and rational use of foods such as citrus will be a major tool in prevention, especially of the chronic and degenerative diseases.

We also increasingly recognize that the ultimate goal of medicine is a social one. The basic objective is to keep man adjusted to his environment as a useful and productive member of society, or, if necessary, to readjust or rehabilitate him. In order to achieve this, medicine must constantly apply the methods of science and investigative research.

Although medicine is only recently awakening to the fact that prevention is of major importance, history tells us that our political leaders have long been aware of this. Benjamin Disraeli declared, "the health of the people is really the foundation upon which all their happiness and all their powers as a state depend." Those who practice preventive medicine must then apply to individuals the knowledge and techniques from nutritional, medical, social, and behavioral science to prevent or retard disease.

In order to better understand the role of nutrition in disease prevention, it is essential to know something of the nutritional status of the American people. Therefore, the highlights of the recently concluded National Nutrition Survey (10), which involved a population of some 70,000 people in ten states, will be reviewed. These data indicate that nutritional problems do exist, even in our generally affluent country. The food supply and nutrition patterns must also be considered as important epidemiological factors in the distribution and determination of disease. Altered nutritional status is one of the major environmental circumstances under which disease may develop and flourish. We must continue to study the interaction of time, place, and person and the role of nutrition in the development of disease. Obviously a knowledge of these factors will also provide the basic information required to prevent development of disease and to maintain health.

The Role of Nutrition in Maintaining Health and Preventing Disease

The World Health Organization defines *health* as a "state of complete physical, mental and social well-being and not merely the absence of disease or infirmity." Modern society further recognizes that the enjoyment of the highest attainable standards of health is one of the fundamental rights of every human being without distinction of race, religion, political belief, or economic or social condition.

Although current expenditures for medical care exceed 7 per cent of the gross national product of the United States, large numbers of people still do not have ready access to continuing comprehensive and quality medical care. Preventive health care receives only scant attention.

Preventive health care is that branch of medicine which has a primary interest in preventing physical, mental, and emotional disease and injury in contrast to treating the sick and injured. Secondarily, it is concerned with slowing the progress of disease, reducing disability, and conserving maximal function. Preventive medicine must focus then on the earliest identifiable phases of the natural history of disease by identifying individuals who are at risk and who become increasingly vulnerable with time. Once risks are identified, every effort must be directed toward reducing them. Here food and nutrition are powerful tools. The proper selection of food to improve nutrition probably offers the best opportunity for improvement of health, not only of individuals but of our nation as a whole (11).

Nutrition and appropriate food selection are recognized as potent

5

forces in public health and preventive medicine; in fact, here may lie the greatest potential of nutrition. Citrus products represent a major contribution to one of the four major food groups and are well justified as a regular component of a balanced diet essential in maintaining health.

THE NUTRITIONAL APPROACH TO PREVENTIVE MEDICINE

A major objective of clinical medicine has been the early diagnosis of disease so that appropriate therapeutic procedures can be instituted promptly before extensive pathology and damage occur. This philosophy is not sufficient for the prime objectives of preventive medicine which emphasize that one need not wait for a disease to develop, even if only in the early state, before an appropriate preventive counterattack is undertaken. Practitioners of the preventive approach recognize that many precursors of disease may be present long before the signs and symptoms appear. The earliest possible identification of disease precursors or risk factors with the implementation of risk-reduction efforts may well be effective in at least deferring or perhaps preventing the disease.

Many of the risk factors or precursors of disease relate directly to diet and food selection. Food and nutrition are therefore key environmental factors in the maintenance of health through risk-reduction programs. The nutritional approach to prevention is emphasized, and the particular place of citrus in a rational nutritional program will be identified. That "we are what we eat" is more than an aphorism, it is a truism.

THE EVALUATION OF NUTRITIONAL STATUS

We have developed a reasonable ability to anticipate disease and to recognize that there may be a sometimes slow and insidious deviation from good health. To pinpoint these changes is a major challenge of preventive medicine. Nowhere is this truer than in the case of nutritional disorders. Alertness to the importance of nutritional well-being may have been dulled somewhat by the fact that the frank deficiency diseases such as scurvy, pellagra, beri-beri, and rickets have largely disappeared from our medical scene and, in fact, have almost become medical curiosities in our hospitals (12). These deficiencies, however, crop up from time to time, particularly in obviously malnourished elderly patients, in chronic alcoholics, or in persons who have subsisted on inadequate or inappropriate diets for long periods of time. The severe stresses of surgery, emotional trauma, or prolonged infection or fever may also enhance the development of nutritional deficiency. Although primary nutritional deficiency due solely to inadequate food intake is rare, it does occur if faulty dietary habits persist. Marginal nutritional deficits are usually not manifested at the clinical level but may occur commonly in relation to such factors as inadequate nutrient intake, poor absorption, decreased utilization, increased nutrient excretion, increased nutrient destruction, and increased nutritional requirements for metabolic reasons. The sequential events in the development of malnutrition are presented in Figure 1 of the Appendix and, whether induced by primary dietary deficiency or by secondary deficiency, lead first to a gradual tissue desaturation of nutrients evidenced by nutrient level alterations in blood, urine, and tissues (Appendix Tables 1 and 2).

As tissue depletion progresses, biochemical lesions may become increasingly manifest by reduction in enzyme activity and altered metabolite levels (13, 14). It should be emphasized, however, that biochemical changes in the blood, like sharply defined clinical manifestations of malnutrition, do not develop in clear-cut and isolated stages but rather in a series of increments in which the time factor is most important. Certainly, blood levels of ascorbic acid both in plasma and in white cells may fall to the vanishing point without overt signs and symptoms of scurvy being manifest (15). This certainly does not mean, however, that a state of "good nutrition" or optimal health exists.

For example, scurvy was the scourge of the long sea voyages of the early explorers, and the disease became rampant after about 100 days at sea. This historical note provides the earliest indication of the time that it takes to deplete the metabolic reserves of ascorbic acid in man. This in no way implies that throughout the 100-day period of progressive ascorbic acid depletion the sailors were functioning optimally or were in "good health"; in fact, "sickness became increasingly common" (28).

Nutritional deficiency is seldom easily discernible; more often than not it is identified as a "gray zone," which adds emphasis to the philosophy of a daily recommended nutrient allowance. Making the daily recommended allowance a "life style" habit is a good preventive nutritional practice.

Ultimately, if inadequate nutrition persists long enough, the classical anatomical lesions or signs of deficiency disease appear (12). It is of interest that complete responses to full nutritional therapy are often slow. Therefore, it is as important to diagnose problems of malnutrition before the disease is fully developed as it is to diagnose appendicitis before the appendix ruptures.

The fundamentals of nutritional evaluation are not significantly different from those used traditionally in clinical patient evaluation (12). They are based on: observing the general appearance of the patient; taking a good medical history; obtaining a careful dietary history, either abbreviated or detailed, depending upon the circumstances; giving a thorough physical examination; and obtaining pertinent laboratory measurements. Finally, and perhaps most important, there is the necessity of thinking of malnutrition and improper food selection as among the many factors that a physician must consider in his attempt to understand the underlying disease process that brings the patient to his office or, more important, by instilling good preventive health practices utilizing the tool of good nutritional practices.

People, Nutrition, and Food

After the air we breathe and the water we drink, our daily food supply is the most important and continuing environmental factor influencing our growth, development, and life itself. The words food and nutrition are frequently used interchangeably, although food, or the nutrients in food, cannot exert nutritional function until eaten, digested, absorbed, and finally converted by the body's metabolic chemistry to be used for all of life's physiological functions. It is also well to remember that there is no single, homogenous eating pattern in the American way of life (16). Food and eating habits are often highly individualized and personal. The kind and type of food, methods of cooking, and patterns of eating vary infinitely from low- to high-income groups, from farm to city, and from region to region. Relatively few foods have universal appeal, but citrus fruits and juices may well be listed in this distinctive category—almost everybody likes them. In general, it cannot be stated that in the United States a region, district, state, or even county has a completely uniform culture concerning food and its use. Food plays a significant part in the ritual of many social ceremonies, including religious ones. Although nutritionists tend to place great emphasis, quite properly, on the nutrient content of food, we must be aware too that the appearance, taste, palatability, the way food is served, and the environment in which it is served may all have important bearings on the acceptance of food and its physiological utilization.

Need vs. Desire for Food

Man has a basic natural urge to eat, to satisfy hunger. In our affluent society, however, hunger satisfaction is not the only drive that causes us to eat or to select the foods that we eat. In general, nature, perhaps unwisely, has left man pretty much on his own regarding what he should eat. Although food satisfies the basic physiologic need to appease hunger, food selection is not instinctive or physiologic. There is no evidence that there is any instinctive or ''master'' direction for one to select the most appropriate foods to insure one's good health. In fact, man appears to have a unique ability to select those things which often have an adverse effect on health, and certainly the excessive use of food has led to the all too common problem of obesity.

One's food habits are formed early in life and are markedly influenced by family and a host of cultural, ethnic, religious, economic, and social factors. These habits are deeply ingrained. There are, of course, many meanings and symbols conveyed by food. Food provides security, and it may be a symbol of power, status, and prestige; it may be used as a reward or punishment. Some foods are associated with special functions, festivals, family rituals and customs, or holidays. A whole set of myths about foods has developed such as, ''fish is a brain food'' or ''fish and milk should not be eaten together.'' Despite the fact that individual food habits are established early, gradual changes are taking place and these will no doubt continue.

Today, more than ever before, people are becoming intensely interested in the kind and quality of foods they eat. There is a desire to learn what foods to eat to stay healthy, what are the most nutritious foods, the hazards of food additives, and the truth about health foods and organic foods. Along with uncertainties have come criticisms and complaints. We are increasingly moving into an era of consumerism in which both the food industry and the government are being asked very difficult questions about the quality of the foods that we buy and eat (17). The current program of food labeling as established by the Food and Drug Administration confirms these concerns (18). We are also seeing a significant growth of food faddism, the development of special health food stores, and the sale of so-called organic foods.

To date, nutritionists have identified some 40–50 chemical substances as nutrients essential to the efficient functioning and health of the body. Most of these can be quite adequately supplied by appropriately selecting readily available foods in the marketplace. Certain basic guidelines have been established which make it very easy for the consumer to select intelligently from the vast array of available foods. The tremendously rapid development of convenience foods and snack foods may have a "diluting effect" on the quality of nutrition, and this will no doubt be an area of increasing surveillance on the part of appropriate agencies. One of the more important guidelines for the kind and quantity of nutrients necessary to maintain health may be found in *Recommended Daily Dietary Allowances*, published by the Food and Nutrition Board, National Research Council, National Academy of Sciences (19, and Appendix). Another and more practical way to determine the necessary nutrients is through the use of the *Basic Four Guidelines*. The philosophy of the basic four approach is that one should select the proper quantity and variety of foods from each of the four food groups each day and handle and prepare these foods so as to minimize losses of nutrients prior to eating. *The emphasis again is on variety and selection from each of the four basic food groups.*

The Basic Four Food Groups

1. The Milk Group

A number of the members of the milk group have universal appeal. Fluid whole milk, skim milk, evaporated milk, and dry milk powder, along with a variety of cheeses and ice cream, are the main foods commonly selected from this important group.

2. The High Protein or Meat Group

This group provides a wide and popular choice of foods, including beef, veal, lamb, pork, poultry, fish, and organ meats. Eggs, dried beans or peas, soybeans, and lentils, nuts, or nut butter may be substituted for a portion of meat in this group. The meat group, along with the milk group, provides the main base for high quality protein in the American diet.

3. The Vegetable and Fruit Group

In this group, variety is of particular importance. It is a very large group and, for simplification, may be broken into three subgroups. It is a recommended common practice to choose one serving of food from each of these three subgroups and then one or more, preferably from the first two subgroups.

Subgroup A.—Deep green or yellow vegetables (such as broccoli, carrots, and sweet potatoes).

Subgroup B.—Citrus fruits and juices, tomatoes, and other fruits rich in vitamin C (such as strawberries, melons, and blackberries) or vegetables (such as green peppers, cauliflower, and asparagus).

Subgroup C.—Potatoes and other fruits and vegetables (such as pineapples, bananas, apples, beets, lima beans, and corn).

Data on consumption clearly indicate that citrus fruits and juices represent a very commonly used subgroup of the vegetable and fruit group (as indicated by an increase in the production of citrus concentrates and Annual Packs, see Appendix).

4. The Bread and Cereal Group

The choice in this group is from whole grain and enriched breads, cereals, a variety of pastas, rice, corn meal, and grits. Cookies, cakes, crackers, muffins, biscuits, pancakes, and waffles also belong in this category.

Generally, as income and economic status decline, and as costs increase, particularly for those items in the first two groups, there is an increasing tendency to select foods from group 4 (the breads and cereals). When such imbalance of food use from the basic four occurs, an increased intake of carbohydrate and a decreased intake of high quality animal protein is the result (20). To make proper ideal use of the basic four food groups as a basis for meal planning and preparation, a variety selection from each of the four groups must be made. Of course, alterations in this procedure may be required based on factors such as food allergies, nutrient intolerance (i.e., lactase deficiency), or a variety of individual idiosyncrasies and economic conditions. Consultation with a nutritionist for appropriate adjustment in the basic four food group selection is suggested.

Oil, fat, and sugar are excluded from the basic four food groups except as they occur naturally in the various foods. Also excluded are the many sources of so-called empty calories such as alcoholic beverages, soft drinks, and candies.

It must not be construed that malnutrition will result if foods are not selected from each of the four food groups in planning the daily diet. In fact, some two-thirds of the world's population seems to get along on a diet emphasizing foods from groups 3 and 4, which provide a wide variety of readily available and more economical foods. Those individuals who are strict vegetarians turn increasingly to legumes such as soybeans, lentils, and dried peas and also rely on other foods, such as nuts, seeds, and whole grain breads and cereals. The lacto-vegetarian diet provides the additional advantage of utilizing milk and related products to provide high quality animal protein; if eggs are also used, the diet may be referred to as an ova-lacto-vegetarian diet. Recent studies have demonstrated that with care and good judgment, it is possible to construct a vegetarian diet that provides the essential nutrients.

Health Foods and Organic Foods

Broadly speaking, there is no such thing as a single health food, although whole milk probably comes nearest to this definition. Still, milk is not totally adequate, and for some it may even be hazardous. Remember, each one of us is an individual with an individual set of metabolic machinery. By and large, health foods are those which have been processed as little as possible. It is well to remember that such foods are subject to labeling laws that govern all foods. To be an informed purchaser you should read and understand the label. In general, if "health foods" are selected they should be adjusted to a variety pattern of food selection, and good meal planning practices should provide a nutritional base comparable to the basic four plan.

The Organic Food Craze

Again, the term "organic food" is a misnomer, in that foods are comprised of organic substances containing, variously, carbon, hydrogen, oxygen, and nitrogen. It is usually understood, however, that "organic foods" have been grown without the use of chemical pesticides or fertilizers and grown on soil that has been treated only with "organic" and natural mineral-containing fertilizers. The principal problem of organic foods becomes one of identification and specification. Who is to know whether or not the food really is "organic," since it is difficult by any measurable analysis to differentiate between the organically grown food and the one produced by customary procedures. Furthermore, the cost of organic foods is generally considerably higher, and although organic food devotees maintain that the taste merits the cost, this is a most subjective matter and hard to prove.

Food Enrichment

The concept of enrichment or fortification of food started more than twenty-five years ago. In a sense, food enrichment became necessary as a part of the changing food habits of the American public. The public's preference for white bread and the necessity of refining cereals to produce white flour, with the consequent loss of nutrients, indicated the need for enriching the flour to insure the maintenance of a desirable and optimal nutrition pattern. The addition of vitamins D and A to a variety of products, particularly milk and margarine, is deemed a sound practice, again to insure nutritional quality. Currently, there is interest in and concern about the enrichment of selected foods with iron, because of the commonness of iron deficiency anemia and the belief that the usual diet may not provide enough iron. As food processing and the preparation of special and convenience foods become more common we will increasingly resort to the enrichment process to ensure nutritional adequacy.

There is little doubt that the application of nutrient additives to processed and refined foods will increasingly come under the jurisdiction and specified limits established by the Food and Drug Administration and its labeling program. One could reasonably ask if it is good nutritional sense to first remove those nutrients inherently present in a food only to add them in a subsequent enrichment process. Food technology is obviously a very sophisticated science which seems to be making food products that consumers will buy, and the food processing and enrichment or fortification procedure is undoubtedly here to stay, but under clearly defined supervision and limitations.

NUTRITIONAL STATUS—U.S.A.

Is there evidence of malnutrition in the United States? The probability that serious hunger and malnutrition exist was brought out in Congressional hearings held as early as 1967 (21). Several extensive reviews have also been published citing nutritional evaluations of a variety of different groups under many different experimental and study situations (22–24). Because of the increasing concern that malnutrition exists, particularly in low-income groups, a ten-state nutrition survey was inaugurated in 1968 and completed in 1970. The results of this survey have been published (10) and merit serious study, particularly for those interested in the epidemiology of malnutrition. It has been pointed out that ''the population studies were not representative of the entire population within a county or state and the survey findings cannot be extrapolated and applied to the over-all population of states from which samples were drawn'' (10).

Some of the major findings in the survey indicated that ''a significant proportion of the population surveyed was malnourished or was at high risk of developing nutritional problems'' (10). The findings further demonstrated that characteristics of malnutrition are often unique to local situations and to specific subsegments of populations being surveyed. This makes it very difficult to provide common nutritional solutions to the different problems that exist from community to community.

The fact that many persons make poor food choices which are largely responsible for their inadequate diets and also often make poor use of their food stamps and the money available for food points up the need for greater consumer education in the area of food and nutrition. Many households seldom used foods rich in vitamin A or vitamin A precursors. Despite the fact that obesity was more common in the adults of low-income groups, the dietary data indicated that there were a substantial number of children and adolescents with caloric and nutrient intakes below the recommended dietary standards.

Of considerable concern was the evidence of poor dental health and that dental caries seem to be associated with between-meal snacks of high-sugar-containing foods such as candies, soft drinks, and pastries. These findings suggest the serious detrimental effects that improper food selection and poor nutrition may have on dental health.

Retardation of growth and development was, in general, more common in lower-income groups. Interestingly, black children generally were taller than white children and were more advanced in skeletal and dental development, indicating a significant racial difference as an important factor influencing growth and the need for appropriate standards specifically for both groups. Obesity as a major manifestation of malnutrition was particularly prominent among black women. In some age groups more than 50 per cent of the adult black women were obese.

The ten-state nutrition survey revealed certain important factors concerning specific nutrients (10). In this survey population there existed a very significant problem of iron deficiency anemia. Low levels of hemoglobin were commonly associated with low levels of serum iron and, to a lesser extent, low levels of serum and red blood cell folic acid. Pregnant and lactating women are significantly vulnerable to poor diet and food habits, and this group of women demonstrated low serum albumin levels, indicating that their protein intake was less than adequate. Because outcome of pregnancy as measured by normal birth-weight infants in good health with fewer neonatal complications is observed to be less than satisfactory in low-income groups compared to the national average and because of an excess of low birth-weight babies in low-income groups, the problem of protein nutriture requires additional evaluation.

The adequacy of vitamin A nutriture indicated special problems for certain groups, such as Spanish-Americans in the low-income ratio states, and, primarily, Mexican-Americans in Texas. It was also noted that "young people in all sub-groups had a high prevalence of low Vitamin A levels." Vitamin A deficiency as a clinical finding was not evident.

Although there was not a major problem of ascorbic acid malnutrition among the general groups studied, "males generally had a higher prevalence of lower plasma ascorbic acid levels than did females and the prevalence of poor ascorbic acid status increased with age."

The summarization of the data derived from the ten-state nutrition survey illustrates the great difficulties in conducting nutrition evaluations among the general population. Improper sample selection and the limitation of the study to a relatively few essential nutrients, while many, many more are identified as essential for good health, loom as important problems which limit interpretation of the data. It was also pointed out that inadequate information is available on the distribution of nutrients in today's food supply.

CURRENT NUTRITION GUIDELINES—RDA

Perhaps the most valuable and at the same time misused nutritional guidelines are the Recommended Dietary Allowances (RDA) developed by the Food and Nutrition Board of the National Research

Council (19). These guidelines are revised periodically, the latest being the eighth edition published in 1974 (see Appendix). The objectives of the RDA deserve re-emphasis because they are so frequently misused. The "allowances are intended to serve as goals for planning food supplies and as guides for the interpretation of food consumption records of groups of people. The actual nutritional status of groups of healthy people or individuals must be judged on the basis of physical, biochemical and clinical observations combined with observations of food or nutrient intakes. If the RDA are used as reference standards for interpreting records of food consumption, it should not be assumed that malnutrition will occur whenever the recommendations are not completely met" (19). It is this latter point that merits special attention, because all too often both the scientific and popular literature have interpreted it to mean that individuals are at nutritional risk of varying degree because their nutrient intake does not conform to the RDA. Compliance with the RDA does not guarantee an adequate nutrition intake nor does failure to comply indicate inadequate nutrition.

The RDA are designed for the hypothetical, perfectly well, "reference" man, woman, or child. Such a mythical man, woman, or child does not exist in reality. In fact, the hypothetical, well individual, or reference man, woman, or child is a nonentity so far as the practicing physician is concerned. Roger Williams has placed great emphasis on the fact that we are "abnormal normal" and that "we have a biochemical individuality that is as distinctive as the individuality of our appearance" (25, 26). This individuality is so distinctive that it is unlikely that any individual will resemble the so-called reference individual referred to in the RDA. These concepts add further difficulty in utilizing the RDA as an interpretive guideline in the evaluation of individual nutritional status. Undoubtedly, more attention will have to be paid to *individuals* and their specific needs. "We shall have to learn why we are such abnormal normals."

Despite these and many other criticisms, the RDA has served as a reasonable yardstick for measuring the adequacy of the nutritional status and will probably continue to do so until some more definitive and better measurements become available.

PUBLIC EDUCATION AND KNOWLEDGE
REGARDING NUTRITION

There is considerable reason to believe that the general public is either generally uninformed about the fundamentals of diet as it relates to good nutrition and health or it is apathetic to this problem. The continued escalating success of "health food" stores, "organic food" sales, and "food fad" magazines and literature indicates no great lack of concern on the part of the public regarding adequate nutrition education but certainly signifies a very high level of misdirection of their interests. Public educators, including nutritionists, must unquestionably assume a high level of responsibility for this unfortunate state of affairs. Basic nutrition education should begin in the home, to be followed and expanded in the public schools at all levels, including an identification of the appropriate facts concerning food and nutrition and their influence on health and the normal physiological development of the individual.

The early impact of improper nutrition education along with the establishment of poor nutritional habits in the pre-school age group bring to mind the importance of the "late effects of early nutrition" and certainly emphasize the long range, adverse health impact of establishing poor food habits early in life and of being misinformed or lacking knowledge regarding the quality of the diet in relation to health.

It is hoped that the family will be reaffirmed as the central focus not only for the preparation and delivery of quality food and nutritious meals but also as a center around which personal health care must be based.

A recent survey undertaken at the suggestion of the Senate Committee on Aging revealed a substantial popularity of certain questionable health practices and beliefs that have been demonstrated to be either fallacious or at best of unproved value. These practices seem to be based not necessarily on faulty beliefs but on the widespread concept that individuals vary greatly in response to treatment, and therefore, "anything is worth a try." People also seem to believe that "if faith in a treatment can work wonders, then any treatment can work." This general ignorance regarding nutrition and health also extends to other areas of public knowledge about health. For example, public education studies indicate that a large percentage of individuals still are not familiar with the very well publicized symptoms and signs of cancer. Only approximately 50 per cent of people questioned could name at least one symptom of diabetes, a very common disease.

A careful monitoring of television programming indicates that in general commercial television has a long way to go to fulfill its public responsibility to educate accurately and effectively about health (27).

Nutritional knowledge is often made more difficult than necessary for two reasons: (a) almost everyone is a self-styled expert in nutrition and ever ready to recommend specific foods, diets, or magic recipes that will provide some miraculous benefit, and (b) there is not enough recognition of the fact that food as such is not nutrition; food only becomes nutritious after it is ingested, digested, absorbed, and the various nutrients utilized in the metabolic mix for growth, development, and tissue repair.

Bizarre advice about foods, special nutrient mixtures, and dietary practices is the trademark of the food faddist, and such information should be refuted with sound scientific fact by the responsible nutrition community at every opportunity.

Nutritional advice to the public, emphasizing the use of a wide variety of foods such as the basic four food groups that will supply the RDA as set forth by the Food and Nutrition Board of the National Research Council, represents sound progress in good nutrition and preventive medicine. This should not imply, however, that these recommendations can be applied indiscriminately or improperly, and it must be recognized that each individual may have special nutritional concerns to which special consideration must be given. This then may require individual evaluation.

Citrus Nutriture

7

ASCORBIC ACID NUTRITURE

Earlier editions of this publication reviewed in great detail the extensive history of ascorbic acid deficiency and scurvy and identified the key chemical, biochemical, and metabolic aspects insofar as they are known regarding ascorbic acid in human nutrition both in health and in disease (1, 2).

For those clinicians who have never seen scurvy in its full manifestations it is perhaps not redundant to record the observations of Kramer, a Hungarian physician, who in 1730 made the following significant comment: "Scurvy is the most loathsome disease in nature; for there is no cure for it in your medicine chests; no, nor in the best furnished apothecary shop. If you can get green vegetables or the juice or pulp of oranges, lemons or citrons you will without other assistance cure this dreadful evil." This statement preceded the observations first reported in great detail in a *Treatise on the Scurvy* published in 1753 by James Lind, a Scottish naval surgeon, who conducted one of the first controlled clinical nutrition experiments in which he demonstrated the value of citrus fruits in the treatment of scurvy. Although citrus was clearly identified as having quite specific and remarkable therapeutic effects, the specific nutrient, ascorbic acid, was not known.

It is an interesting commentary on the vagaries of human nature and the impediments of bureaucracy to note that it was not until 1795, nearly half a century later, that the British Admiralty issued an order which required a daily ration of citrus juice for all members of

19

the Royal Navy. During that half century almost 200,000 British sailors are said to have died of scurvy. Even today, in our presumably more enlightened society, we often move with pathetic slowness in translating the fruits of our basic and clinical research into practical application for the individual and at the bedside.

Scurvy—Ascorbic Acid Deficiency and Physiologically Sensitive Groups

Scurvy in its most fulminating clinical form has been reported in association with every war in history. Certainly circumstances of adverse climate, living conditions, and stress associated with battlefield or shipboard conditions seem to enhance the opportunities for bringing forth the characteristics of scurvy in its classical form (28).

It is interesting that although citrus fruits and juices and ascorbic-acid-containing vegetables are readily available in the marketplace, and despite the fact that there is a considerable advocacy for the use of synthetic vitamins, including ascorbic acid, scurvy has not disappeared, although it is rare. The problem of diagnosis may be more difficult because doctors fail to obtain an adequate dietary history. Certainly ascorbic acid deficiency is not at all uncommon among the elderly, the indigent, alcoholics, individuals with malabsorption syndromes, and, unfortunately, many long-term institutionalized patients for whom cooking losses in preparation and service of food for large numbers of people may substantially reduce the ascorbic acid content of the diet. Strangely enough, ascorbic acid deficiency and even scurvy appear to be on the increase in the younger pediatric age group despite our nutritional knowledge and the ready availability of orange juice. It is also becoming evident that latent forms of ascorbic acid deficiency, manifested by very low serum and white blood cell levels of this vitamin, are all too common. The latent aspects of ascorbic acid deficiency have been more clearly identified in autopsy studies on infants which showed that scorbutic lesions appeared ten times as often as the disease was diagnosed in infants on the basis of clinical signs. This certainly stresses the concerns expressed for the prevalence of "hidden" ascorbic acid deficiency, particularly in infants.

It appears that, as with many nutrients, there exists a spectrum of nutritional adequacy with respect to ascorbic acid (29). The interrelationship of ascorbic acid levels and tissue saturation, utilizing different parameters of measurement, are indicated in Table 1.

Certainly blood levels of ascorbic acid may fall to zero without clinical manifestations of scurvy, but, on the other hand, serum plasma levels of ascorbic acid in excess of 1 mg. per cent are required to achieve from 60 to 80 per cent tissue saturation (30). The white blood cell levels of ascorbic acid are generally much higher than plasma levels and tend to diminish and ultimately disappear substantially after serum plasma levels reach zero. What index and what level of tissue saturation should the clinical nutritionist use as a measure of adequacy of ascorbic acid in the diet?

TABLE 1. Interrelationship of Ascorbic Acid Levels

% Tissues (saturation)	% Test dose (ascorbic acid in urine)	Plasma level (mg. %)	Buffy coat (mg. %)	Ascorbic acid intake (mg. %)
Saturated	60–80	1.0	27–30	100
Saturated	20–60	0.4–1.0	15–20	40–100
½ Saturated	10	0.2–0.4	12–15	10–15
¼ Saturated	5	0.05–0.2	5–10	5–7

This remains a hotly debated subject made more heated by the pharmacological, macromolecular doses of ascorbic acid recommended by some.

Metabolic Role of Ascorbic Acid

It is of considerable interest that only certain species, such as man, monkey, flying mammals, and the guinea pig cannot synthesize ascorbic acid (1, 2). Obviously then, these species depend totally on dietary sources for sufficient amounts of ascorbic acid to prevent deficiency and scurvy. The multiple functions of ascorbic acid in the animal body have been reviewed in detail in earlier editions (1, 2), and only the highlights of its metabolic functions will be identified here.

As a key nutrient in the synthesis of collagen, ascorbic acid has been identified in the reaction by which proline is hydroxylated to form hydroxyproline, a key component of collagen. A number of other hydroxylation reactions also depend on ascorbic acid. It also plays a significant role in folic acid metabolism (to be discussed later). Another index of the importance of ascorbic acid in the problem of anemia is indicated by its specific role as a reductant of the ferric ion upon its transferal from plasma transferrin to liver ferritin.

Classically, ascorbic acid has been demonstrated to be effective in wound healing, which may relate to its role in collagen synthesis (31). The relationship of ascorbic acid to stress and adrenal cortical change during stress is of unquestioned importance, although the mechanism of action is not clearly understood.

An interesting new parameter has developed which has given further insight into the amounts of ascorbic acid that may be needed by man living under controlled environmental circumstances and under very carefully supervised nutritional and metabolic conditions (30, 32–36). By labeling ascorbic acid with radioactive C_{-14}, isotope studies have been conducted in a number of laboratories to determine the size of the body pool of ascorbic acid which thus permits its actual utilization by healthy adult men to be accurately measured. Such studies have provided the first clear index to the "basal" needs of ascorbic acid and indicate that there is a mean utilization of 21.5 mg. per day of ascorbic acid with a rather large standard deviation of 8.1 mg.

These isotopic metabolic studies have also provided significant information about the metabolic products of ascorbic acid which in man appear to be oxalic acid, ascorbic acid, and ascorbic acid-2-sulfate. These also appear to be the primary storage form of ascorbic acid in animals. In young, healthy, male volunteer subjects, studied under controlled environmental and dietary conditions, the ascorbic acid pool size was 2–3 gm., and the turnover half-time of ascorbic acid was about 20 days on intakes of about 100 mg. per day. Similar pool sizes and turnover rates have been reported in other studies. The first symptoms of mild scurvy appeared in these experimental subjects when their body ascorbic acid pool size had been reduced to about 300 mg. The rate of repletion of ascorbic acid was a zero order process and generally proportional to the level of daily ascorbic acid intake.

Unfortunately, a general review of these very sophisticated studies may raise more questions than are finally answered. While they have confirmed what the body pool size of ascorbic acid is, and have reasonably confirmed the levels needed to prevent scurvy, they have provided little additional information regarding the metabolic and biochemical functions of ascorbic acid at the molecular, enzymatic, or cellular level. We do not have sufficient information to identify precisely any coenzymatic role for ascorbic acid and may consider it useful only as a general antioxidant. The great specificity of ascorbic acid in preventing and treating scurvy and in metabolic reactions such as biological hydroxylation and in the metabolism of folic acid mitigate against this hypothesis. Undoubtedly, ascorbic acid may serve in biochemical and metabolic functions at enzymatic levels that are not yet identified. As indicated earlier, the significance of increased requirements of ascorbic acid to meet the substantial biochemical changes that occur in stress indicate it has a primary, although yet unidentified, role as a specific metabolic nutrient. We have only begun to explore the biochemical role of this most interesting vitamin.

Stability of Ascorbic Acid in Fresh and Cooked Foods

Consumers of citrus fruits and juices are interested not only in the ascorbic acid content of these products but also in its stability during storage. The generally recognized lability of ascorbic acid upon exposure to oxygen and heat is particularly associated with certain other elements such as iron and copper. Ascorbic acid in freshly harvested citrus products occurs chiefly as L-ascorbic acid, which is the reduced form of the vitamin. When subjected to alkalinity, exposed to oxygen or heat, particularly in the presence of metallic ions, it is oxidized readily to dehydroascorbic acid. This latter compound possesses biological activity almost equal to that of ascorbic acid, but it is relatively labile and is further easily converted to 2,3-diketogulonic acid, which does not possess ascorbic acid activity. This sequence of reactions is portrayed in Figure 1.

Most of the ascorbic acid data published in food tables are the results of analyses for L-ascorbic acid. It is difficult to compile representative values for the ascorbic acid content of foods in the published literature because a number of investigators have determined and reported the reduced (L-ascorbic) form and the dehydroascorbic acid form of the vitamin, both of which have approximately equivalent biological activity. Some of the data have indicated the sum of the active forms without indicating how much of each was present, and a few studies have included diketogulonic acid as part of the total ascorbic acid content, which, of course, is a falsely elevated value with respect to biological activity. The principal reason for this lack of uniformity is that the two most widely used chemical methods for ascorbic acid analysis do not measure these compounds separately, and, in fact, they measure different things.

The oxidation reduction properties of ascorbic acid are utilized in the methods that employ 2,6-dichlorophenolindophenol, which is an oxidizing agent and a dye. The extent to which a solution of this dye is de-colorized by ascorbic acid is utilized to determine the content of the reduced form of the vitamin in foodstuffs.

The other widely used method for the chemical analysis of ascorbic acid involves the coupling of dehydroascorbic acid with

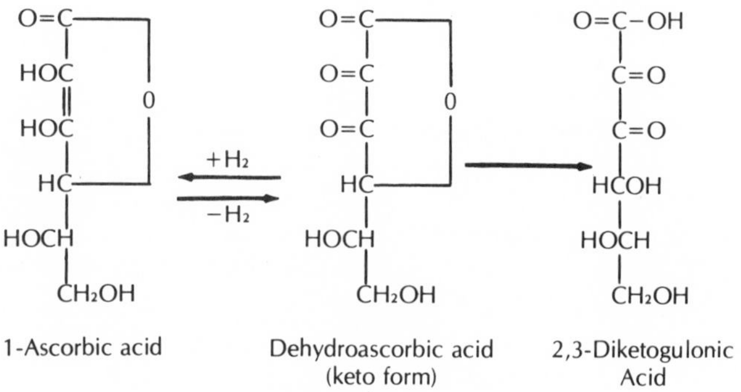

1-Ascorbic acid   Dehydroascorbic acid   2,3-Diketogulonic
                       (keto form)   Acid

FIGURE 1. Degradation of ascorbic acid.

2,4-dinitrophenylhydrazine under controlled conditions to give a characteristic red-colored osazone which is then measured colorimetrically, the intensity of the color being proportional to the amount of ascorbic acid present. It should be emphasized that this method requires the conversion of the reduced form of ascorbic acid (the naturally occurring vitamin) to the dehydroascorbic acid form which is then measured. Generally speaking, this method of ascorbic acid determination reflects total biological value and is generally higher than the previously mentioned dye method.

These two methods have been used independently and in combination to determine the stability of ascorbic acid in citrus products under a great variety of storage circumstances. A recent study utilizing the method which includes both ascorbic and dehydroascorbic acids concluded that ascorbic acid was actually remarkably stable under controlled laboratory circumstances of substantially elevated temperatures, provided that oxygen and trace minerals were kept in minimum contact with orange juice. The results of these studies (37) are summarized in Appendix Tables 8 and 9.

Although the above experiment was conducted under the somewhat artificial circumstances of the laboratory, many other studies concerning the stability of ascorbic acid in a variety of citrus juices indicate a remarkable stability under a wide variety of storage conditions. There is little doubt that the acidic nature of citrus and citrus juices protects them very substantially against the destructive forces that oxidize and destroy ascorbic acid (38, 39).

In general, ascorbic acid in fresh citrus fruits is exceedingly well protected during storage and is quite stable. The nutrients in whole citrus fruit are also well protected by the peel.

The story regarding the ascorbic acid stability in cooked foods is substantially different, and a great many studies have been reported (40, 41). In general, these studies indicate that there is a substantial variation from day to day in the amount of L-ascorbic acid provided by the foodstuffs offered, particularly from the steam counters of cafeteria lines and in large-scale institutional food preparation and service. To underline the significance of the loss of ascorbic acid, associated particularly with institutional cooking, in only three of the ten periods studied did the average L-ascorbic acid content of the foods served meet the RDA for ascorbic acid. Home cooking may also result in losses of ascorbic acid, not only from the heat, metal containers, and cooking time, but also by the leaching of the ascorbic acid into the cooking water (40).

The foods with the largest contribution of ascorbic acid per serving are citrus fruits, fresh strawberries, tomatoes, raw cabbage, broccoli, cauliflower, brussels sprouts, and spinach.

It appears that the largest degradation of ascorbic acid in canned and glass-packed citrus juices occurs primarily during the first few days of storage and is associated with the rapid disappearance of the minimal free oxygen remaining in the cans. Subsequently, the rate of loss is only about one-tenth that in this early period.

In summary, the acidic characteristic of citrus products and the "gentleness" and high level of food technology applied in the processing of citrus fruits appear to minimize the oxidative destruction of ascorbic acid in these products.

FOLIC ACID

Folic acid is a yellow, crystalline compound widely distributed in nature and particularly in deep green, leafy vegetables and such organ meats as liver. It exists in a variety of forms such as the free vitamin folacin, conjugated with glutamic acid in a peptide linkage, and in a formylated state. The physiologically active forms of folic acid are reduction products, tetrahydropteroyl glutamic acids. Primarily, folic acid coenzymes function in the transfer of single carbon units in a number of intracellular metabolic processes, particularly in the synthesis of purine and pyrimidine ribotides and deoxyribotides and in amino acid interconversions. Folic acid itself appears to be readily absorbed by the gastrointestinal tract, while its conjugated forms are enzymatically degraded to the monoglutamate form prior to absorption. Certain conjugase inhibitors may be present in some foods which block the action of the enzymes that liberate free folic acid from the conjugated forms (42).

Tetrahydrofolic acid plays a key role in the various chemical reactions in which folic acid participates. The folic acid reduction process is catalyzed by an enzyme (folic acid reductase) and triphospho-pyridine nucleotide. Ascorbic acid plays a prime role in keeping folic acid in its reduced form by protecting the reductase enzyme.

It is important also to note that scurvy patients who are given test doses of folic acid show very little increase of folinic acid in the urine until 5 or 6 days later, again indicating the key role for ascorbic acid in activating folic acid in the reduced form.

There is also some evidence indicating that vitamin B_{12} deficiency may induce a secondary deficiency in the folic acid coenzymes either by reducing the amount of folic or folinic conjugase converted to folic or folinic acids or the amount of folic acid coenzymes formed (43). Ascorbic acid deficiency may interfere with folic acid metabolism in a similar manner.

A further interlocking of key factors associated with anemia is indicated by the fact that a deficiency of iron may have an adverse effect on folic acid metabolism since formimino transferase is an iron-containing enzyme. Thus, a deficiency of this enzyme may interfere with the formation of formimino tetrahydrofolic acid. This suggests that iron deficiency, particularly common in pregnant women, may accentuate the megaloblastic effects of folic acid deficiency.

Determination of Folic Acid in
Biological Materials (44, 45)

The content of folic acid in foods and biological tissues can be determined by the application of several microbiological assays. The microorganism most commonly used is *Lactobacillus casei*, which measures folic acid, its reduction products, the di- and triglutamates of folic acid, and N-methyl tetrahydrofolic acid, which is the major component of serum. Unfortunately, there is no single method that will accurately determine all of the folic acid metabolites. Generally, in order to measure the higher conjugases of folic acid, especially in foods, the food extract must be treated with a conjugase enzyme preparation before the determination is made.

Interpretation of Folic Acid Nutriture (46–52)

It must be emphasized that a deficiency of folic acid may cover a very wide spectrum of biochemical and physiological changes before all the manifestations of megaloblastic anemia appear. In estimating the adequacy of folic acid intake, it is important to obtain an adequate dietary history, particularly focusing on those foods which may contribute significant amounts of folic acid to the diet, such as orange juice or green leafy vegetables. Methods of cooking are, of course, important in view of the destructive influence of heat on folic acid in foods. Actually most foods, with the exception of citrus, contain little or no free folic acid. This then points to the need of the liberation of folic acid from the conjugate during the digestive process and, as indicated earlier, there may be inhibitors in certain foods which impair this liberation process (53–55).

The appearance of formimino glutamic acid in the urine after a test load of histidine has been proposed as a measure of folic acid deficiency. During pregnancy this particular metabolic abnormality, suggesting folic acid deficiency, is quite commonly observed.

Man has body stores of folic acid sufficient for about 120 days before severe signs of folic acid deficiency become evident. These body stores are actually very small, approximately 5 mg. of folic acid.

In view of the rather recent observation of a significant level of folic acid in citrus products, particularly orange juice, and because of the significance of citrus in the diet as one of the key representative members of the basic four dietary pattern, this aspect of folic acid evaluation requires special comment.

Hoppner, Lampi, and Perrin (56) determined the free and total folïc acid activity in 162 foods available on the Canadian market. They utilized the *L. casei* method for both the free and conjugated forms of the vitamin. It had been previously noted that the addition of ascorbic acid to the basal medium used for the assay procedures protected against the loss of the labile forms of folic acid. They also observed the protective effect of ascorbic acid during analysis, which was reflected in both the free and total folic acid activities that they reported.

The folic acid contents for oranges and grapefruit in μg. per 100 gm. of fresh weight were 24.0 plus or minus 8.3, and 10.8 plus or minus 3.3, respectively (this represented total folate activity).

Dong and Oace (57) have also studied the folic acid distribution in fruit juices, utilizing three microbiological methods for both free and conjugated folic acid. Using *L. casei*, the total folic acid contents for orange and grapefruit juices as μg. per 100 ml. was 52.6 plus or minus 6.5 and 21.1 plus or minus 1.7, respectively. More than 95 per cent of the total biologically active folic acid in citrus juices was due to methyl folate. They conclude that orange and grapefruit juices are excellent sources of dietary folic acid.

Is the folic acid in orange juice well utilized? Nelson et al. (58) studied the normal subjects to evaluate the absorption of both folic acid and ascorbic acid from orange juice and also from solutions containing synthetic sources of these vitamins. An elegant procedure using a triple lumen tube with a 30 cm. sampling segment permitted the estimation of these water-soluble vitamins absorbed from the proximal jejunum. The results showed no significant differences in the absorption of folic acid and ascorbic acid whether from orange juice or synthetic sources. Folic acid in orange juice appears to be well utilized.

Streiff (59) has also identified orange juice as a particularly rich and practical source of folic acid and emphasizes its use, since, as he points out, the cooking or processing commonly applied to most foods may destroy some 60–95 per cent of the folic acid. (This percentage of loss does not apply to citrus products and hence makes them an important food source of folic acid.) Again using the *L. casei* method, no polyglutamate of folic acid was found either in the pure orange juice or juice pulp. The pulp contains some folic acid but not as much as the juice on a weight basis, and the orange peel has a very low folic acid level. Streiff concludes that "five to seven ounces of orange juice will supply approximately 100 to 150 µg. of folic acid which is well within or above the minimum daily requirement of folic acid for adults" (59). This would also represent a substantial percentage (at least 25 per cent) of the folic acid RDA.

Other studies of the folic acid content of the total mixed diet indicate that American diets on the average may contain 52 plus or minus 14 µg. of free folic acid activity per day, and after digestion with conjugase, which liberates folic acid from the conjugated forms, the total folic acid activity increases to 184 plus or minus 67 µg. per day (60). In the Canadian study, based on the apparent per capita disappearance of foods in Canada in 1966 and the recently determined folic acid values for foods, the average daily intake is approximately 140 µg. of free folic acid which is increased to 210 µg. of total folic acid activity per person per day after treatment with folic acid conjugase. This represents a folic acid intake less than the RDA. Again it should be emphasized that these values cannot reflect the vagaries of dietary selection or the impact of severe cooking losses and that they point to orange juice as an important daily food source for folic acid to provide a significant part of the RDA.

Folic Acid Depletion Associated with
Anti-Convulsant Therapy

Low serum folic acid levels, which may be associated with megaloblastic anemia, may develop when anticonvulsant drugs (i.e., diphenylhydantoin) are used during prolonged therapy. This finding has been reported in two separate studies (61, 62). In one report, twenty-seven patients with seizure disorders were evaluated with respect to serum folic acid, iron, iron-binding capacity, and the hemagram. It was noted that dietary intakes of iron, folic acid, and ascorbic acid were adequate, but despite this, folic acid serum levels were extremely low. One must question the adequacy of folic acid intake reported in this study as 50 µg. per day; this is certainly less than the RDA of 400 µg. per day, and probably near the minimal requirement.

It was observed that, "The fact that folic acid and its derivatives are 'convulsant' greatly increases the significance of the drug in-duced changes in folate metabolism in epileptic patients, and strengthens the hypothesis of a relationship between anti-epileptic and anti-folate metabolism" (62). It was further noted that, "it is not without significance that a substance which has convulsant properties may also when in short supply, result in mental symptoms."

THIAMIN AND RIBOFLAVIN (63–65)

Thiamin and riboflavin, vitamin B complex members, are vital components of enzyme systems that are particularly relevant to nutrient metabolism. The general details of their importance in nutrition, their site of metabolic action, and their contribution to the physiological well being of man have been reviewed in the earlier editions of *Citrus Fruits in Health and Disease* (1, 2). Relevant here is the possible contribution that citrus fruits may make to the nutritional intake of these vitamins as used in a regular daily allowance of at least one serving (6 oz.) of orange juice.

Thiamin participates in a particularly significant coenzyme which functions in carbohydrate metabolism in the decarboxylation of alpha keto-acids and in the utilization of pentose in the hexose monophosphate shunt. Of particular significance is the role that thiamin plays in relation to caloric need and the metabolism of carbohydrate to yield calories. Although it has been noted that dietary fat spares the thiamin need to some extent, this reduction does not appear to have great significance in practical nutrition and diet planning. By and large, approximately 0.33 mg. of thiamin per 1000 kcal. fulfills the requirement and 0.4 mg. per 1000 kcal. is sufficient to meet an RDA that allows for individual variation. In the United States, a current base of recommended dietary allowances considers that 0.5 mg. of thiamin per 1000 kcal. will maintain adequate thiamin nutriture.

With the general utilization of thiamin as part of the enrichment mixture for many products, particularly cereal and flour, the problem of meeting the daily nutritional needs for thiamin has been greatly eased. Also, one aim in our nutritional pattern is toward a lowered caloric intake which should also reduce moderately the recommended daily need for thiamin. Generally speaking, the fruit and vegetable group provides thiamin in foods with lower caloric values than the cereals and meat and can make a significant contribution to the daily thiamin recommended allowances. The thiamin and riboflavin contents of citrus products are listed in detail in Table

10 of the Appendix. Based on the RDA for thiamin, which in general reflects the caloric intake of various groups of people, and ranges from 1.0 to 1.5 mg. per day, the amount found in 6 oz. of 12.8° Brix orange juice will provide nearly 12 per cent of the recommended dietary allowance. This may be of particular significance in view of the common practice of including citrus products, and particularly orange juice, in the daily dietary program.

There is evidence of an increased need for thiamin during pregnancy and lactation; in particular, the thiamin content of human milk is influenced by thiamin intake.

POTASSIUM (66)

There is no specific RDA for potassium since it is assumed that an adequate intake is assured by the fact that it is so widely distributed in foods and that its usual intake based on a varied diet will range from 2000 to 4000 mg. per day. Potassium is primarily an intracellular ion and, in fact, occurs in the greatest concentration of any mineral within the cells of the body.

Substantial amounts of potassium may be excreted in the urine and lost from the body, particularly during diuretic therapy associated with the treatment of hypertension. Patients who are digitalized vigorously and who are also receiving diuretics may even with a mild potassium depletion run the risk of digitalis intoxication.

Citrus juices offer one of the most favorable sources of potassium with respect to the potassium-sodium ratio and also in regard to their total potassium content (see Appendix). Very few foods provide as high a potassium-sodium ratio as does orange juice, and certainly very few foods provide comparable levels of potassium in a nutritional blend that is so continually well accepted by the patient. The excellent palatability, the ready availability, and the economical cost of orange juice make it an ideal adjunct to insure against excessive potassium losses in patients receiving diuretics. For example, a 6 oz. serving of orange or grapefruit juice will provide approximately 335 and 277 mg. of potassium, respectively. One study (66), in which fifty-four elderly patients were treated with diuretics for three months, demonstrated that citrus fruits given daily successfully prevented symptoms of hypokalemia. Most clinicians agree that for most individuals being treated with the usual doses of diuretics, the dietary sources of potassium and especially citrus fruits are sufficient to maintain electrolyte balance.

If one relies wholly on diet to maintain normal potassium levels, one should be aware of the signs and symptoms of potassium depletion. The presence of this syndrome will require, of course, more specific therapeutic management with potassium supplements (67). Fortunately such circumstances are rare. Potassium depletion may be manifested by impaired neuromuscular function, which may vary from mild weakness to overt paralysis. Abnormalities of heart function may be manifest with disturbed ECG patterns, conduction defects, and an altered sensitivity to digitalis. There also may be an inability to concentrate urine appropriately and an occasional depression in renal filtration rate. In addition to diuretic agents, certain of the mineralocorticoids may effectively result in the increased loss of potassium which may be related to the increased renal tubular reabsorption of sodium. Potassium depletion may also be a consequence of primary hyperaldosteronism caused by an adrenal cortical adenoma or of secondary hyperaldosteronism with adrenal cortical hyperplasia often accompanied by hypertension.

Serum concentrations of potassium normally range between 130 and 180 mg. per liter. Potassium is primarily an intracellular ion, and a normal range of serum potassium does not guarantee that there may not be a significant deficit of potassium. Potassium body deficits of as much as 8–16 gm. may occur before the serum level of potassium is reduced below 120 mg. per liter. Alternations in the electrocardiogram, including a prolongation of the Q-T interval and a broad and flat T-wave with a depression of the S-T segment, indicate myocardial conduction defects reflective of potassium deficiency.

In summary, potassium deficiency is not likely to be encountered under normal circumstances of dietary intake or in the absence of unusual therapeutic medications or disease which might enhance potassium excretion. When potassium deficiency is present or threatens, citrus fruits and juices offer excellent nutritional sources of potassium, and they are also nearly devoid of sodium.

SODIUM—THE ROLE OF CITRUS IN LOW-SODIUM DIETS

Patients with hypertension and hypertensive cardiovascular disease with congestive heart failure are usually directed to maintain low-sodium diets; such patients must be educated to understand the sodium content of commonly used foods and drinking water and what foods to delete entirely from the diet (68–70).

Furthermore, the person who plans and prepares the food for a sodium-restricted diet must know the sodium content of the various foods in the diet and the amounts of the other constituents that may influence the health and nutritional status of the patient or individual. To assist in these matters the American Heart Association has recently published a guide which suggests various foods for diets that are restricted to 1 gm., 500 mg., and 250 mg. of sodium per day. Each of these diets specifies at least one daily serving of oranges or grapefruit and suggests that the amounts can be substantially greater if no specific caloric restrictions are imposed. Fresh, peeled citrus fruit or fruit juices have negligible quantities of sodium and can be used generously in sodium-restricted diets, the only limitation being again the number of calories permitted.

For individuals who like salty foods or who are in the habit of salting their foods liberally, salt-restricted diets are most unpalatable. The use of a few drops of lemon juice certainly enhances the palatability of many foods, and the diet is often greatly improved not only by the good flavor of citrus fruits but by their generally appreciated aromatic characteristics.

Fortunately, the normal renal tubule has a tremendous capacity to reabsorb sodium and prevent excess sodium losses even on very rigidly restricted sodium intakes. The usual adult intake of from 8 to 18 gm. of sodium chloride per day greatly exceeds the amount of sodium required to maintain sodium balance. With normal renal function the sodium requirement is certainly less than 300 mg. per day. Many nutritionists and pediatricians have viewed adversely the high sodium content of many commercially prepared infant foods, and recommendations have been made to reduce the salt content of foods designed specifically for infants.

PECTIN

Pectin is a general term commonly used for any of the class of pectic substances which comprise approximately 0.2–1.0 per cent of the succulent parts of plants and a wide variety of fruits and vegetables, including citrus. The diet of Western man, with its many refinements and many new types of food, is relatively low in roughage. It is becoming increasingly evident that for optimal nutrition, the diet should contain a reasonable level of these nonabsorbable complex carbohydrates, which provide bulk. It has been postulated that one of the possible reasons for the increasing incidence of cancer of the colon is that our diet has become increasingly refined and very low in bulk. Pectins could perform a useful function in supplying such bulk. The carbohydrate structure of pectic substances is related to galacturonic acid which is analogous to galactose in chemical composition except for an acid group in place of the terminal hydroxyl of galactose. These units are strung together in long chains; the acid COOH group is a side chain of the cyclic form of the carbon unit, and methylesterification of this carboxyl group takes place to a varying degree. The length of the pectin chains may be quite variable, but in general they are long enough to function as colloids with water binding an outstanding characteristic. The pectic substances in fruits generally have a high content of the methylester of the carboxyl group, and the pectin in oranges has about 80 per cent of the maximum methoxyl content possible. Studies conducted to demonstrate the cholesterol-lowering effect of pectin have utilized pectin by incorporating it into a number of baked products, such as cookies, bread, rolls, etc. Using this technique, it has been possible to get as much as 50 gm. per day of pectin in the diet, which resulted in substantial lowering of blood cholesterols in experimental subjects.

In many ripe fruits, soluble pectic substances occur between the plant cells also. Commercial pectin is the soluble substance industrially derived from these pectic substances. Pectin NF indicates that the product meets the standards for pure pectin set by the National Formulary. Since the intestinal tract of man does not contain enzymes that permit their digestion and breakdown, the pectic substances provide no calories. In general, pectic substances do not disintegrate below the size of colloids in the upper portion of the gastrointestinal tract and hence retain very high water-binding characteristics. This water-binding function gives a high moisture content to the food and intestinal contents and presumably favors good digestion with bulk. Some of the pectic substances in the cell walls of food are converted to relatively soluble pectic substances, and those may be important for the improved digestion and availability of other nutrient components of the food. Ripe fruit, for example, contains substantial quantities of these solubles, and the softening of the fruit as it ripens accompanies this pectic change. Certainly, all of the pectic substances are not converted to the more soluble forms, probably due to the very large size of the molecule and possibly to the presence of hemicellulose, insoluble mineral salt groups in the molecule, or a combination of these. In the lower intestinal tract, however, where the microbial population is very great, digestion of these pectic substances is more extensive. It is presumed that these end products of the digestive process produced by intestinal microorganisms are advantageous to the pH, which is, in turn, advantageous to flora of the colon.

DIETARY FIBER

Dietary fiber has recently been labeled "the forgotten nutrient." It is well known that fiber promotes regular "elimination." However, recent scientific evidence is now establishing a new and perhaps more vital role for dietary fiber—its potential in preventing the onset of a variety of gastrointestinal diseases (194). The typical diet of the Western world is highly refined and lacking in bulk, and research studies now suggest a correlation between the low fiber content of the diet and the increased incidence of gastrointestinal disease, including cancer of the colon. In rural Africa, where the fiber content of the diet is high, conditions such as constipation, diarrhea, hiatal hernia, diverticular disease, and cancer of the colon are rare. These diseases, on the other hand, are common in the Western world (195).

Although the evidence is far from conclusive, many gastroenterologists are now recommending that the Western cultures return to the natural laxatives provided in foods such as wheat bran, whole grain cereals, legumes, and fresh fruit and vegetables. The positive effect of dietary fiber, including pectins, on regular elimination is a result of high water binding capacity and increased bulk. Fiber from cereal bran and from fresh fruits and vegetables (in particular carrots, mangoes, apples, brussels sprouts, and citrus products, especially oranges and grapefruit) perform equally well as bulk agents (196). Bran, unfortunately, is difficult to obtain and is frequently unacceptable to the patient's taste and palate. On the other hand, citrus products (oranges and grapefruit) provide both acceptability and sufficient fiber to improve bowel habits. They are also generally available at a favorable economic cost. Perhaps a new health slogan could begin "an orange or grapefruit a day. . . ."

THE CITRUS BIOFLAVONOIDS (71, 72)

Bioflavonoids, once designated as vitamin P, are a group of organic substances possessing the basic structure of a flavone. Bioflavonoids are widely distributed in nature as pigments in flowers, fruits, tree barks, and vegetables. The nutritional values for man of the bioflavonoids hesperidin, obtained from oranges, and naringin, from grapefruit, have not been established. Although a great many studies have been conducted on these compounds, there is yet no convincing evidence that they are required dietary nutrients or have any specific physiologic function. Continuing research interest is evident, however, particularly with hesperidin, and a wide variety of therapeutic benefits ascribed to hesperidin continue to be reported. Studies reporting evidence for a favorable effect of bioflavonoids on minimizing capillary fragility and permeability in several animal species have been reported. These findings have not been confirmed in studies with man.

Physicians, coaches, and trainers of athletes have used bioflavonoids to treat a wide variety of athletic injuries. Such studies are very difficult to quantitate or to control and measure accurately but, subjectively at least, the use of bioflavonoids is reputed to promote more rapid recovery from injury. In planning conditioning programs for athletes, it has been suggested that 300–900 mg. or more of citrus bioflavonoids in divided doses be given daily to reduce the degree of superficial bruising injuries. No adverse side effects have been reported, and the so-called loss of time and medical care of injured athletes is reported to be significantly reduced. Studies of this kind are very subjective.

Currently, the use of citrus bioflavonoids in treating athletic injuries is being substantially expanded in amateur and professional baseball, boxing, football, and track teams. These programs include dietary supplementation with citrus bioflavonoids throughout the training period and the season schedule.

The absorption of hesperidin and other citrus bioflavonoids has been well demonstrated by in vivo biological tests and by the identification of their urinary metabolites. There is little apparent relationship between the water solubility of the flavonoids and their absorption, metabolism, and physiological activity except for their parenteral use in animals where solubility is an obvious factor. Metabolic by-products of hesperidin and other citrus bioflavonoids have been identified, indicating that they are subject to metabolism, and metabolic end products have been identified in the urine. The sum of these experiments provides evidence for the absorption as well as the metabolic cleavage of the flavonoid molecule.

A number of bioflavonoid materials have been studied for their effect on capillaries and on minimizing capillary fragility (73). A number of procedures have been utilized to determine the degree of capillary fragility. Apparently, the therapeutic rationale of combining bioflavonoids with ascorbic acid or other therapeutic agents is based on the premise that capillary integrity should be maintained. It has been suggested, and a number of experiments have been cited to support the suggestion, that citrus bioflavonoids in conjunction with ascorbic acid appear to enhance the efficacy of other therapy and aid in controlling such factors as infection, stress, and nutritional deficiency, even in cases in which capillary weakness is not manifested. The substantial details of these experiments have been summarized and reported elsewhere. Szent-Gyorgyi, who has been a pioneer in the flavonoid investigative area, feels that the chelate formations of the flavonoids hold the key to understanding their biological function and that flavonoids represent "one of the most exciting, broad and hopeful fields of biological inquiry" (149). Their ultimate value remains to be proven.

Nutritional Status of Four Age Groups

Orange Juice in Pediatric Nutrition

Orange juice continues to be one of the most commonly recommended food sources of ascorbic acid by pediatricians probably because it is a reliable source, practical to use, readily available, of modest economic cost, and generally well accepted by infants and growing children. It is difficult to understand why scurvy is ever seen in infants and small children, but the fact remains that in the five-year period of 1956–1960, 226 teaching hospitals in the United States reported admission of 713 infants and children with scurvy. More recent statistics indicate that scurvy continues to be a problem (74–77). Part of this may be related to the fact that bottle feeding is practiced far more commonly than it once was. Although the human being is unable to synthesize ascorbic acid, the lactating female is able to concentrate it in her milk, and breast-fed infants are thus protected from deficiency. Bottle-fed infants, on the other hand, may receive only 3–6 mg. of ascorbic acid per day on pasteurized cow's milk formulas, and unless this vitamin is added to the diet, the average plasma ascorbic acid levels in the infant may become low. The earliest clinical manifestations of ascorbic acid deficiency are apathy, loss of appetite, and increased irritability. Since these are not uncommon symptoms in small infants, ascorbic acid deficiency may not be considered until there is overt tenderness of the lower extremities and joints and even hemorrhages of the skin and mucous membranes. Interestingly enough, iron deficiency anemia is frequently associated with ascorbic acid deficiency (78–81). For the most part, the failure of infants to receive an adequate amount of ascorbic acid relates to poor nutritional education of the parents or a lack of understanding that certain milks and milk formulas may be low in that vitamin. Surprisingly, scurvy is no less prevalent in Florida than it is in the rest of the country, even though that state is the home of citrus fruits. This emphasizes the need for adequate education of both the public and the medical profession; it also implies some serious gaps in our health care system.

To prevent infantile scurvy and to assure a normal rate of growth and normal health, orange juice supplement may be started during the first month of life, providing 30 mg. of ascorbic acid per day,

TABLE 2. RECOMMENDED SCHEDULE FOR INTRODUCING ORANGE JUICE INTO THE DIETS OF INFANTS

Age (weeks)	Amount orange juice (teaspoonfuls)	Amount boiled water dilution (teaspoonfuls)
2	1	1
2½	2	2
3	3	3
3½	4	4
4	5	5
4½	6 (1 oz.)	6 (1 oz.)
5	7	6
5½	8	6
6	9 (1½ oz.)	6
6½	10	6
7	11	6
7½	12 (2 oz.)	6

the amount commonly received by the breast-fed infant. This is usually given in the form of orange juice. Table 2 is a recommended schedule for introducing orange juice into the diet of infants in the age range of 2–8 weeks.

There are some, such as Whelen et al. (82), who believe that natural orange juice is a better source of ascorbic acid than the synthetic vitamin. They recommend 1 daily teaspoonful of orange juice diluted with an equal amount of boiled water, starting at 2 weeks of age. The amount is increased to twice weekly by 1 teaspoonful of each until 1 oz. of orange juice and 1 oz. of water are reached. Thereafter, only the juice is increased until, at 2 months of age, the infant is receiving 2 oz. of orange juice diluted with 1 oz. of water. At 1 year of age, the infant receives 3 or 4 oz.

of orange juice daily. Premature infants, because they may be born with low stores of vitamin C, should be given ascorbic acid supplements of up to 100 mg. daily after the first or second day of life.

Others have also published suggestions that natural sources of ascorbic acid are superior to the synthetic form of this vitamin (83–85). This point of view is controversial and poorly substantiated by evidence.

In view of the desirability of implanting the preference for healthful foods, it is recommended that orange juice be instituted as part of the nutritional pattern for infants as indicated above. However, one must consider that some children do not appear to tolerate orange juice satisfactorily. There are those, for example, who spit up the juice and who do not seem to like it. Some babies may even appear to exhibit gastrointestinal upsets after taking orange juice. Fortunately, these situations are infrequent; it would, however, be unreasonable and unwise to continue feeding orange juice under circumstances which might implant in the child a distaste for a product which, if delayed in its use to a more suitable age, would be well tolerated and enjoyed.

"Allergy" or Intolerance to Orange Juice in Infants

In actual fact, a very small minority of infants are upset by orange juice. However, when feeding problems associated with the use of orange juice do develop, it is realistic for the pediatrician to advise an appropriate temporary substitute for orange juice. This discontinuance of orange juice then becomes a matter of practicality and is generally not based on a genuine food allergy or food intolerance. Again, common sense dictates that one does not persist in a practice which may cause discomfort, dislike, or unreasonable difficulties.

It is far more important for the pediatrician to educate the mother to the fact that citrus products, particularly orange juice, are natural and wholesome foods and are practical, abundant, and relatively economical sources of ascorbic acid as well as other important nutrients, and that unquestionably, at a later point in the child's life orange juice will be welcomed as an important ingredient of a well-balanced diet. The philosophy to establish is that all individuals, including infants and small children, should be taught to get the maximum amount of vitamins, minerals, and other essential nutrients from a varied diet, starting as early as possible in infancy. Vitamin supplements may be used as just that, namely to provide a "filling of the gap" when a normal spectrum of food intake may be less than desirable for a variety of reasons.

Nearly all foods, particularly those containing significant levels of protein, are potentially allergenic. Some of these food intolerances are not genuine allergies in the usual antigen/antibody sense, which is the scientific fact to be evaluated when a patient is thought to be allergic to a food. Intolerances to foods (not genuine allergies) may arise because of enzyme defects which lead to an inability to deal in a normal way with various food constituents. Individuals with lactase deficiency, for example, cannot utilize lactose adequately. Most commonly, when food intolerances occur it is generally agreed that tests using elimination diets may be more practical than skin tests and more informative in elucidating the problems of such sensitivities or intolerances.

There is evidence to suggest that "allergenicity" to orange juice (i.e., skin or respiratory allergies) may be related to chlorogenic acid. This is a very common organic acid found in many plant materials, including oranges where it tends to be concentrated primarily in the peel or in the fibrous tissue immediately adjacent to the peel and the fruit. The normal processing of orange juice should exclude all but an insignificant amount of chlorogenic acid in orange juice or orange juice concentrate.

Ratner et al. (85) and Joslin and Bradley (86) have reported that allergenic type reactions to orange juice, whether manifest by gastrointestinal hyperactivity or skin reactions, are quite rare in infants. It has been suggested that such reactions may be attributed to the small amounts of peel oil in the juice which may cause pseudoallergic dermal and gastric irritations. Minimizing the pressure on the orange when squeezing it will reduce the amount of peel oil in the juice. Joslin and Bradley (86) also comment that the gradual introduction of orange juice into the infant's diet, starting at 2 weeks of age with ¼ oz. diluted with an equal amount of water, greatly minimizes any tendency for intolerance to the juice. Since true food allergies are predominantly due to an antigen/antibody reaction related to the absorption of food proteins, foods that are generally rich in protein, such as eggs, milk, fish, and nuts, are the most commonly identified and potent food allergens. Cow's milk, because of its common usage, particularly in the diet of the young, is perhaps the food that has been most extensively studied in relation to its allergenicity.

Although it appears that the so-called allergenic potential of orange juice is greatly exaggerated and may reflect only mild intolerances manifest by spitting up the juice, it again makes sense to discontinue the use of orange juice for a time and return it for another trial when the child is older.

Lawrence and Hawley (87) have also compared the so-called allergenic reactions of 114 infants to chilled orange juice with comparable reactions to a commercial instant breakfast drink containing synthetic ascorbic acid and to a control solution simulating orange juice. The infants were studied from the age of 2 weeks to 3 months. Skin rashes were equally evident in all three groups, including the control group, thus questioning the validity of "allergic reaction" that is commonly attributed to the production of rash in children by orange juice. In this study of 15 infants who appeared not to like the preparation given them, only 3 received pure orange juice.

Ascorbic Acid Requirements for Children

As indicated previously, while overt scurvy in children is rare, it does occur all too often and raises the question of whether or not they actually receive enough ascorbic acid in their daily diets, not only to prevent scurvy, but to insure proper bone formation and normal growth and development, particularly during the rapid growing period.

The Food and Nutrition Board, National Academy of Sciences, National Research Council, recommends a daily dietary allowance of 40 mg. of ascorbic acid for the age range of 1–10 (19). Infants from 0 to 1 have an RDA of 35 mg. of ascorbic acid. Vitamins are not infrequently prescribed by physicians and are also purchased "over the counter" by individuals. The consumption of synthetic sources of vitamins is probably higher in North America than anywhere else in the world. Although Americans have probably the highest standard of living and generally produce a surplus food supply, one wonders if the general population suffers from a lack of vitamins. This philosophy may be undergoing considerable change in view of the rapidly developing "megavitamin" concept (to be discussed elsewhere). Actually, however, we have remarkably little information on the vitamin intake of infants and children either from food or from synthetic sources.

Mott, Ross, and Smith (88) made a special study of the intake of vitamins C and D, which were added to some foods in which they are not normally present, to determine if, for example, there was any evidence of hypervitaminosis with respect to vitamin D. Since ascorbic acid is also commonly prescribed for infants, both its intake and that of vitamin D were estimated in a population of 1200 infants attending the health centers that were being evaluated. The populations studied included individuals from low-income, high-income, and low- to moderate-income levels, as well as a group from a separate, adjoining municipality having a broad type of population covering all income levels but predominantly the "average level."

With regard to vitamin D, an analysis of the data demonstrated that about 1 per cent were getting more than 2000 IU, 93 per cent were getting between 400 and 2000 IU daily, and 6 per cent were getting less than 400 IU daily, which is, of course, below the RDA. Of the group studied, 70 per cent received more than 400 IU from diet only, and 79 per cent received more than 400 IU from a vitamin supplement only. With regard to ascorbic acid, 85 per cent of the infants were receiving more than 30 mg. of this vitamin daily while 15 per cent received less; 63 per cent were receiving over 50 mg. daily from diet and vitamin supplements, 56 per cent were receiving more than 30 mg. daily from diet only, and 57 per cent received more than 30 mg. daily from synthetic vitamin supplements only.

Although there is no evidence of harm from hypervitaminosis C, 63 per cent of the infants studied were receiving more than 50 mg. daily, which represents an unnecessary expenditure of family funds considering that the RDA of ascorbic acid for infants and children can quite adequately be met by the appropriate use of orange juice.

Of greater concern is the fact that 15 per cent of infants received less than 30 mg. of ascorbic acid while 4 per cent received only insignificant amounts of this vitamin. In such cases these infants were receiving less than 1½ oz. of orange juice daily and none or an inadequate amount of vitamin supplement containing ascorbic acid.

This study points up the fact that adequate nutrition education is of particular importance especially in the home setting where the parents are the principal providers of food and have a major responsibility for insuring an adequate nutrient intake. Unquestionably, the home is the most important setting for the maintenance of health and the prevention of disease. For the most part, it is the center for the care of individuals during the most sensitive and fragile physiologic and psychological periods of life, involving primarily the newborn, the very young and growing children, the pregnant woman, and the aged. Unfortunately, the home often becomes a focus for isolation, and nutritional problems may be hidden there and may be further enhanced by the nutritional ignorance of the individual responsible for providing food. In addition, there are obviously many social and economic pressures which lead to the disruption of the home setting and subsequent improper and oftentimes inadequate nutrition.

THE NUTRITIONAL STATUS OF ADOLESCENTS

All too often the adolescent teenager "falls through the cracks" of health care supervision, being a bit too old for the pediatrician and a bit too young for the internist. Needless to say, the growth period beginning just before puberty and continuing through maturation into adulthood often gives rise to significant health problems and is certainly associated with a host of biochemical and endocrine changes along with very significant alterations in body mass and composition. The age period from 12 to 18 years is of particular importance and requires special attention in the provision of adequate nutrition for satisfactory growth and development. It must also be remembered that many girls in this age bracket become pregnant, which further increases nutritional demands, and, unquestionably, poor nutrition is a very important factor in the large incidence of low-birth-weight infants with elevated neonatal and infant mortality that is associated particularly with very young mothers. The National Nutrition Survey (10) directed its concern toward this age group and substantial numbers were included in the survey.

An extensive survey of teenagers in Iowa provides a wealth of information concerning the adequacy of their nutrition (89). These data suggest that high school students have highly individualized dietary habits which do not necessarily reflect either the economic status of their families or the recommendations of their parents. Dietary "faddism" is frequent, and a sizeable number of students, especially those who skip breakfast, have significantly less than a desirable intake of ascorbic acid which is reflected in lower serum levels of this vitamin. It was also shown that sound nutritional practices depend not only on supplying adequate amounts of the important essential foods but also on the avoidance of excess quantities of other foods that may produce adverse health results. Particularly mentioned is the excessive use of "sources of empty calories" and a remarkably high consumption of foods that are known to be associated with elevations of serum lipids, particularly serum cholesterol. Other studies have also shown that the nutrients most apt to be low in teenage diets are iron, calcium, and ascorbic acid (23). Adolescent girls seem particularly prone to poor dietary habits "principally because of social pressures, misconceptions and general ignorance concerning appropriate normal maturation and knowledge concerning a well balanced diet" (89).

SOME MAJOR NUTRITION–HEALTH PROBLEMS AFFECTING ADULTS

The White House Conference on Food, Nutrition and Health had a panel which addressed itself to the nutritional problems of adults, particularly in an affluent society, with an emphasis on the development of degenerative diseases of middle age. Certain general conclusions were reached. It was considered that the overconsumption of calories along with under-exercise led to obesity which represents a major problem of malnutrition which is in turn associated with other major health problems. The "atherosclerotic cardio-vascular diseases" were also recognized as the major contributors to morbidity and mortality, and while "a causal relationship between diet and atherosclerotic vascular disease remains unproved," there is much indirect evidence to suggest that diet modifications resulting in a reduction of blood lipids may prevent or retard these diseases. It was further recognized that hypertension involving an estimated 21 million Americans is a major health hazard. Although the cause or causes of hypertension remain unknown in approximately 80–85 per cent of the cases, obesity is a major risk factor that is frequently associated with high blood pressure. The restriction of salt intake is beneficial for most individuals with hypertension and "evidence has been accumulating that high intakes of dietary salt from infancy onward may be an important factor in initiating and aggravating hypertension particularly for those with a family history of hypertension and those who already have the disease."

The panel further noted that the excessive use of alcohol, with its direct damaging effect on the liver and general health, as well as its impact on the family and social structure, is a problem of major magnitude. The current per capita consumption of alcohol in the United States indicates that from 10 to 20 per cent of total caloric intake is from this source and represents a significant proportion of "empty calories" in the diet.

Diet and Coronary Heart Disease

A joint policy statement has been issued by the A.M.A. Council on Foods and Nutrition and the Food and Nutrition Board of the National Academy of Sciences, Natural Research Council (98). This statement reidentifies atherosclerosis as the major health problem in America with 660,000 Americans dying each year from heart attack and about 171,000 of these dying before the age of 65 (99). It is significant that almost all epidemiologic experimental and clinical investigations have identified a series of risk factors which significantly increase susceptibility to coronary heart disease (100–107). Elevations in plasma lipids (especially plasma cholesterol), hypertension, heavy cigarette smoking, obesity, and physical inactivity are included in this list of risk factors. The risk of developing coronary heart disease is positively correlated with increasing levels of cholesterol in the plasma (100). It is estimated that about one-third of American men and a less definitely known proportion of women consuming their usual American diet maintain plasma cholesterol levels at or above 220 mg. per 100 ml. It is also clear that the level of plasma cholesterol in most people is influenced by the character of their diet which may contribute cholesterol from the foods they eat or from the ingestion of increased amounts of saturated fat. Plasma cholesterol levels may be lowered by restricting dietary cholesterol and replacing sources of saturated fat in the diet with sources of unsaturated fat. It is also noted that elevation of plasma triglycerides is reflected in an increased risk of coronary heart disease (102, 103). Plasma triglycerides can be reduced through dietary manipulation, particularly by restricting the intake of carbohydrate and especially the simple sugars, such as sucrose.

In summary, the Joint Council report points out that the overall level of plasma lipids in most American men and women is undesirably elevated and focuses on the need for measures which will lower plasma cholesterol. It is recommended that plasma lipids be determined as part of a routine health maintenance physical examination and that such measurements should be made in early adulthood so that appropriate preventive intervention measures may be initiated, particularly in those individuals falling into high risk categories on the basis of their plasma lipid levels. Care must be taken to assure that dietary management is based on sound nutritional principles and includes the intake of foods which contribute all of the essential nutrients. This should be accomplished with relative ease, utilizing ordinary foods, readily available, and reasonably priced. It is highly appropriate to note the role of citrus products of all kinds as an important part of the dietary management of patients with hypercholesterolemia. Citrus products represent a most liberal source of ascorbic acid which has been shown to have a favorable effect in reducing plasma cholesterol levels (to be discussed). In addition no citrus fruit or juice contains cholesterol or fat.

Since a North American male has about one chance in five of developing clinical coronary heart disease before age 60, mostly in the form of myocardial infarction, it is evident that sound nutritional and diet modifications represent important preventive measures. The major point to be made with regard to nutrition is the importance of modifying the diet within sound nutritional limits so as to lower plasma cholesterol and plasma triglycerides.

Citrus Nutrients: Their Influence on Cholesterol Levels

It has been known for some time that citrus pectin, as well as other fruit pectins, administered orally, significantly reduces blood serum cholesterol levels (108–10). Diets supplemented with 15 gm. of citrus pectin per day had a cholesterol-lowering effect which was apparent within 3 weeks. Further studies have demonstrated that increasing the dietary intake of citrus pectin in the range 25–50 gm. per day improves the cholesterol-lowering effect of pectin. It is, of course, difficult to incorporate these larger levels of pectin into the normal diet without first incorporating pectin into such products as bread, biscuits, and other baked products. It appears that the addition of pectin to a basal diet containing cholesterol increases the excretion of fecal saponifiable and nonsaponifiable lipids and decreases the absorption of dietary cholesterol. Evidence that ascorbic acid may play a role in cholesterol catabolism was indicated by the observation that ascorbic-acid-deficient guinea pigs develop atherosclerosis; it was further suggested that the formation of the fatty deposits on the inside of arteries could be reversed by restoring adequate levels of this vitamin to the diet. Rabbits that were fed cholesterol-containing diets showed increased levels in the tissues and increased urinary excretion of ascorbic acid even though these animals (which can synthesize ascorbic acid) had not been given the vitamin. After feeding cholesterol, ascorbic acid levels decreased, suggesting that it has a significant role in cholesterol catabolism.

Gradually, an interesting web of evidence indicating a relationship among ascorbic acid, cholesterol metabolism, and atherosclerosis is being developed. Soviet scientists have published on the relationship of atherosclerosis and ascorbic acid for a number of years. Although their first experiments were conducted with monkeys, more recent studies have been directed toward the relationship of ascorbic acid to atherosclerosis in man.

Spittle (111, 112) has recently reported a study using 58 healthy controls and 25 patients with atherosclerosis. Serum cholesterol levels were measured in each group for 6 weeks; ascorbic acid therapy was then administered at a level of 1 gm. daily and cholesterol levels determined for a further 6-week period. No other dietary restrictions were imposed. The results indicated that in the control group of individuals under the age of 25, cholesterol levels tended to fall after ascorbic acid administration. There was, however, remarkably little change in the age group 25–45. After the age of 45 there was no consistent pattern resulting from the administration of ascorbic acid, and some individuals actually showed a rise in serum cholesterol. Patients with atherosclerosis who were given ascorbic acid also demonstrated an increased serum level of cholesterol; it was suggested that this rise represents an increased mobilization of cholesterol that had been deposited in the arteries. Support for this contention is derived from the results of several studies with animals.

Sokoloff et al. (113, 114) have studied the effect of ascorbic acid on serum lipids in both animals and man. In atherosclerotic patients, ascorbic acid as used in these studies had no effect on serum cholesterol, although it did tend to lower triglycerides toward normal and to enhance the activity of lipoprotein lipase.

A particularly interesting observation compares the status of ascorbic acid nutriture of cigarette smokers and nonsmokers (115–17). Here the ascorbic acid status of 14 cigarette smokers and 14 nonsmokers was evaluated before and after saturation for 6 days with

2.2 gm. of ascorbic acid. The smokers initially had lower blood levels of ascorbic acid and a lower urinary excretion after a 1.1 gm. test dose of the vitamin as compared to the nonsmokers. These differences disappeared after the saturation and desaturation period. It would seem, therefore, that the cigarette smokers initially retained more ascorbic acid, suggesting a lower nutritive status with respect to this vitamin. It has been suggested that atherosclerosis may, in part, represent a long-term deficiency or unsatisfactory nutritive level of ascorbic acid the result of which permits cholesterol to accumulate in the arterial walls and possibly causes changes in other fractions of the tissue lipids. This concept of deficiency clearly does not represent the traditional nutritional deficiency concept; other metabolic factors may be involved which require clarification.

The mechanism of the cholesterol-lowering action of ascorbic acid in man has not been explained. In guinea pigs with a latent ascorbic acid deficiency, the rate of cholesterol catabolism to bile acids is slowed, and there is a pronounced reduction in cholesterol turnover (118). This can be reverted to normal by resaturating the tissues with high doses of ascorbic acid.

Other studies with guinea pigs have also demonstrated that cholesterol accumulates in the blood serum and in the liver when a chronic, latent ascorbic acid deficiency exists (119–21). It has been indicated that this is due to a decreased rate of transformation of cholesterol to bile acids in the liver of animals deficient in ascorbic acid. A direct correlation has been demonstrated between the ascorbic acid concentration in the liver and the rate of cholesterol transformation to bile acids.

What does stress have to do with the development of coronary heart disease? And how does stress relate to an interaction between ascorbic acid and cholesterol in the metabolism of these substances? (See discussion on stress.) Anxiety and certain personality characteristics appear to be associated and may be demonstrated to precede coronary heart disease, particularly angina pectoris, with greater frequency than one expects to find in healthy control samples (106, 107). Life dissatisfactions and environmental stress have also repeatedly been found to be more prevalent in patients with atherosclerotic heart disease. An interesting set of personality traits, such as the Type A personality, and behavioral characteristics called "the coronary prone behavior pattern" is increasingly identified in association with clinical coronary heart disease. The question is whether the behavioral and personality risk factors increase the chances of coronary heart disease by elevating the traditional risk factors (such as blood pressure or cigarette smoking) or do they work through some more basic biochemical mechanism at the cellular level, influencing the so-called stress syndrome which in turn relates to a metabolic interrelationship such as the ascorbic acid–cholesterol interaction. It is a most interesting challenge to attempt to integrate these somewhat intangible behavioral personality characteristics with the still unsettled status of the biochemical data base which relates stress, cholesterol, and ascorbic acid to the development of atherosclerotic coronary heart disease.

The "Coffee Habit"—A Risk of Heart Attack?

A number of factors are associated with an increased risk of heart attack: elevated blood lipids, hypertension, cigarette smoking, lack of physical activity, and obesity. It would seem, in fact, that there is much to support the lament that "Everything I enjoy in life is either illegal, immoral, or fattening." A recent addition to the list of coronary risk factors, and a practice which provides evident enjoyment for many, is the daily consumption of many cups of coffee. A number of studies have been conducted recently which purport to support the concept that coffee consumption is related to the risk of heart attack (122–25).

The most recent report (125) provides data which suggest "a positive association between coffee consumption and acute myocardial infarction—from a multipurpose survey of 12,759 hospitalized patients, including 440 with a diagnosis of myocardial infarction. In comparing those who drink coffee to those who drink no coffee, the risks of infarction among those drinking one to five or six or more cups of coffee per day are estimated to be increased by 60 and 120 per cent, respectively. The association could not be attributed to confounding by age, sex, past coronary heart disease, hypertension, congestive heart failure, diabetes, smoking or occupation, nor could it be explained by the use of sugar with coffee." Interestingly, this study reported that, "There was no positive association between tea drinking and acute myocardial infarction."

Despite these incriminating data, the authors concede (125) that the link between myocardial infarction and coffee drinking is still very much of a mystery and does not permit the conclusion that coffee consumption is a cause of heart attack. Most epidemiologists believe also that conclusive evidence in support of a theory should be obtained by a prospective study in which all of the evidence is accumulated before the onset of a disease. The retrospective study reported (125) is also in marked conflict with the conclusions of several prospective studies, including the well-known Framingham study.

Needless to say, additional information will be necessary to ascertain whether or not coffee can be incriminated as a causative factor in heart attacks. If one is in doubt or concerned about coffee drinking, it may be reasonable to suggest an orange juice break instead of a coffee break; there is still something to enjoy without fear of heart attack—orange juice.

NUTRITIONAL ADEQUACY AND ASCORBIC ACID DEFICIENCY AMONG THE ELDERLY

Although classical nutritional deficiencies are not commonly seen in "acute care" hospital populations in the United States, nutritional inadequacy is common among the elderly. Cases of moderate to severe scurvy continue to be reported most commonly in elderly men who live alone and who do not prepare adequate meals, or who live on subminimal diets (90). The diets of such individuals tend to consist of very easily prepared foods such as bread and butter or sandwiches of various kinds, with tea and coffee. The isolation and lonely life style strongly favor the development of nutritional deficiencies, and since the dietary patterns of many elderly people do not include an adequate amount of citrus products, ascorbic acid deficiency is certainly one of the most common problems noted.

Again, scurvy must be thought of before it can be diagnosed and one must be alert to this possibility when the chief signs and symptoms are pain, lethargy, anorexia, mental depression, small bruises on the limbs, anemia, and extravasation of blood into the tissues. Swollen, tender, and bleeding gums with the development of loose teeth is very common in scurvy. The capillary fragility test with the production of petechial hemorrhages may be noted after the application of a blood pressure cuff. A dietary history will, of course, immediately reveal a deficit of foods containing ascorbic acid. A substantial number of case studies from hospitals both in this country and in England, particularly, point up the seriousness of ascorbic acid deficiency, either overt or minimal. The appearance of scurvy among the elderly admitted to our hospitals probably represents only the "tip of the iceberg," since it is a much more common nutritional problem for the elderly than is generally appreciated. Although the more acutely ill patient may be admitted to the hospital, these not infrequent case reports identify the possibility of a substantial prevalence of clinically undetected or neglected ascorbic acid malnutrition in the elderly population. The fact that slightly more than 10 per cent of the population of the United States is over 65 years of age emphasizes the potential seriousness of this nutritional problem. Further, we have an ever growing geriatric population, and, with the increasing economic squeeze, it becomes more difficult for the elderly person to achieve a good diet and completely adequate nutrition. It is estimated that hunger and malnutrition affect older people more than any other segment of our population. It is believed that as many as 8 million elderly citizens subsist on diets that are insufficient for optimum health, and due to inflation this number is increasing rapidly. Since the cost of food is the second most expensive item for the elderly, ranking only behind the cost of housing, malnutrition may become a serious problem. The lack of nutritional "know-how," the emotional stress related to living in loneliness and isolation usually with recent loss of a loved one or companion, lack of mobility, and inadequate financial resources are additional obstacles to achieving an adequate level of nutrition. Surveys of the dietary patterns of the elderly frequently indicate that they have been living on coffee, tea, doughnuts, and a complete spectrum of other cheap, tasty foods that are high in sugar, starches, and perhaps fat, but often very low in other essential nutritional elements. All too often the elderly subsist on the "tea and toast" diet.

Preliminary results of a long-term study by investigators at the Gerontology Research Center of the National Institutes of Health (NIH) indicate that as many as one-fifth of those not taking vitamin supplements have abnormally low levels of these nutritional essentials. The NIH team finds these results especially surprising since the study group is comprised of well-educated individuals who can obtain adequate diets. These findings again emphasize the necessity of making good nutrition and balanced food selection a habit. Unfortunately, poor dietary habits may be more easily accepted than good ones.

Another factor that mitigates against an adequate intake of citrus, which certainly could satisfy the need for ascorbic acid at a very low cost, is that the dietary patterns of most elderly people were established at a time before citrus products were commonly available at an economic cost. Most of these individuals grew up in an era when oranges and grapefruit were delicacies served only at festive holidays. It is evident, therefore, that the implantation of preference for citrus, and particularly for orange juice, was not made then and hence is not part of their present daily dietary pattern despite the current ready availability, palatability, and modest cost of a 6-oz. serving of orange juice which would generously supply the daily nutritional needs with respect to ascorbic acid.

Studies of elderly patients who have been institutionalized for chronic medical care or for care of the aged have shown them to have very little fresh fruits or fruit juices in their diets and to have a high incidence of ascorbic acid blood levels well below the range considered appropriate for optimum nutrition. Studies have also shown that in addition to the poor dietary intake of ascorbic acid there may be excessive destruction of this vitamin in the gastrointestinal tract, particularly in the elderly.

Andrews, Letcher, and Brook (91) have reported significant decreases in the white blood cell concentration of ascorbic acid in the elderly during the winter months and have further confirmed that the ascorbic acid status of elderly residents of institutions was often considerably lower than that of those living at home. A more recent study involving a 17-month trial of ascorbic acid supplementation in elderly people living in a home for the aged revealed that it was necessary to supplement the diet with 40–80 mg. of ascorbic acid daily before the vitamin levels of the white cell became normal. There was also a marked individual variation in response, supportive of the concept of biological individuality postulated by Williams (25).

Studies of ascorbic acid deficiency in the elderly have also been conducted in Ireland where a level of 30 mg. of ascorbic acid daily is used as the RDA as established by the British Medical Association (90). In this study, 65 per cent of the lower-income elderly subjects examined had an intake of ascorbic acid below the 30 mg. per day level; 25 per cent of the upper-income elderly subjects had diets that were similarly deficient. Despite these deficits, no case of clinical scurvy was seen among the subjects examined. In this connection it was pointed out that it is necessary to distinguish between the amount of ascorbic acid needed for tissue saturation and that needed for protection against scurvy. Full tissue saturation achievement is variously estimated between 50 and 100 mg. of ascorbic acid per day, while protection against scurvy may be provided by as little as 10 mg. per day. Although the majority of the elderly subjects in this study received enough ascorbic acid to protect against scurvy, not enough was provided for tissue saturation. It is suggested that low ascorbic acid levels in the elderly may be a contributory factor to the general lethargy, aches and pains, and fragility of the blood vessels frequently found in older persons. This suggestion is of course difficult to substantiate.

A study of the dietary ascorbic acid intake in the United Kingdom provides information indicating that about one-quarter of households have ascorbic acid intakes that average less than 30 mg. per person per day, the level recommended by the British Medical Association Committee on Nutrition to provide a good margin of safety. It was further noted that as many as 5 per cent of the households may have ascorbic acid intakes below 20 mg. per person per day. These problems are accentuated during the winter months when fresh fruits and vegetables are generally less available and more expensive, but ascorbic acid nutriture improves during the spring and summer. These studies indicate that ascorbic acid nutriture may be a serious problem and that a significant number of households and an ever greater proportion of individuals (particularly the elderly) may have an ascorbic acid intake that is more or less continuously below the recommended level (92).

It is evident from these and similar studies that it is most difficult to ascertain with accuracy the actual consumption of foods and specific nutrients either by households or by individuals within the household. With regard to ascorbic acid, it is even more difficult to estimate with any degree of accuracy the actual level of intake, partly because of individual food preferences of the members of the household, but perhaps more important because of the variability of losses of ascorbic acid that occur during cooking. Certainly the data that have been obtained on cooking show that loss of ascorbic acid, particularly in institutionally prepared foods, is quite significant and results in markedly reduced intakes of the vitamin.

Special Nutritional Concerns during Illness

As might be anticipated, the elderly individual with a history of improper and often inadequate food and nutrient intake may be at added risk due to improper nutritional status when exposed to a variety of illnesses. Decreased serum levels of ascorbic acid are often associated with chronic infection, postsurgery conditions, and chronic inflammatory diseases, especially if these are sufficiently severe or prolonged. Since chronic diseases are of particular concern and are very common among the elderly, nutrition looms as an extraordinarily important supportive measure, requiring emphasis on a balanced and adequate nutritional intake during such periods of illness.

Illness must certainly be considered a form of stress which may be an important factor in altering the requirement for and metabolism of ascorbic acid (to be discussed separately).

Another area of concern not uncommon in the elderly is the problem of alcoholism. Alcoholics frequently exhibit low serum levels of ascorbic acid (also folic acid) and manifestations of ascorbic acid deficiency.

Osteoporosis continues to be a major problem of the elderly, and the favorable influence of citrus juices with their acid pH and metabolic alkalinizing effect suggests their utility as a nutritional aid in the continuing management of this difficult problem (93–95).

Gastrointestinal bleeding is also a significant medical problem for adults. Ascorbic acid has been demonstrated in a number of studies to exert a favorable effect in the management of such disorders by reducing bleeding tendencies (96, 97).

Nutrition and Health Problems

NUTRITIONAL AND METABOLIC ASPECTS OF OBESITY (126–31)

Obesity involves a significant excess of stored fat in relation to other bodily components. In the United States it is estimated that 20 per cent of the population may be considered overweight, that is, 10 per cent above their ideal body weight, while about 10–15 per cent are significantly overweight, i.e., 15–20 per cent overweight. Arbitrarily, obesity may be defined as a condition in which the individual is more than 25 per cent above desirable weight for height and body build and this extra weight represents an excess of stored fat. It is estimated that about 7 million people are so seriously overweight as to represent pathological obesity and that they may be considered "caloriholics." In general, the proportion of fat in relation to total body weight increases with age. In lean, young adults approximately 14 per cent of the body weight is fat, while 25 per cent of the body weight is represented as fat in clinically normal but sedentary men of normal weight at age 55. This probably represents a general replacement of muscle mass with fat as aging progresses.

It is now recognized that much adult obesity has its origin in childhood patterns (132). Obesity originating particularly in infancy leads not only to more fat in each adipose cell but more seriously to a marked increase in the actual number of such cells. The fat cell in the obese is approximately twice the size of the adipose cell in the nonobese. Studies concerning the number and size of fat cells suggest that the total number of these cells becomes fixed in late childhood. Excessive nutrient intake from that point on merely increases cell size. Conversely, weight reduction of a fat adult with an excessive number of fat cells merely converts a fat man into a thin fat man with a continued potential for adding fat back to the fat cells.

There is no doubt that obesity represents an increased hazard to health. Although as an isolated entity it may not be a major risk factor in coronary heart disease until it exceeds 25 per cent of normal weight, obesity is closely associated with diabetes mellitus, particularly of the maturity onset type, and with elevation of blood pressure. The accompanying elevated levels of serum triglycerides, and often cholesterol associated with diabetes mellitus, represent a serious increased risk of the development of coronary, cerebrovascular, and renalvascular disease as well.

Some Metabolic Abnormalities in Obesity (126, 129)

In addition to the increased number and size of fat cells associated with obesity, insulin levels may be two to five times normal in the obese individual and may rise higher than normal during the absorption of carbohydrate and protein. These increased insulin levels are considered to be a manifestation of increased insulin resistance in obese persons, which to some degree negates the biological effectiveness of insulin and thus requires more to be secreted in order to gain an equivalent physiological effect. The cause of this insulin resistance is not known.

Fat turnover in the obese individual is slower during starvation, and obese individuals have a lowered lipolytic effect when certain lipolytic hormones such as growth hormone, glucagon, or adrenalin are administered. Again there is no clear explanation for these abnormalities (126, 129).

Despite these interesting metabolic and endocrine alterations, it is difficult to identify a specific defect, other than caloric imbalance, with an excessive caloric intake over output to explain the cause of obesity. There is also little doubt that the level of activity is an important environmental factor in the development and maintenance of obesity. Obese individuals have been repeatedly shown to expend from one-sixth to one-third of the physical activity commonly demonstrated by thin people engaged in comparable activities (133, 134). The obese individual appears to be significantly hypokinetic in his life style.

Management of the Obese Individual

There is no magical or easy solution to weight reduction. No single program will work for everyone, and unfortunately very few seem to work for anyone. Not only is losing weight a difficult job but it requires eternal vigilance and diet and exercise control to prevent recurrence of weight gain. There is no doubt that food has come to have important social and psychological value for many individuals who seem unable or unwilling to sacrifice the pleasurable sensations of eating despite the various physical, emotional, and health hazards of being obese (135).

Practical Applications of Nutrition in Weight Reduction

Tables of desirable body weights for men and women published by the Metropolitan Life Insurance Company (see Appendix) serve as a reasonable guideline and provide a goal for weight reduction programming (136, 137). It is highly important to establish a reasonable rate of weight loss, and a long-term reasonable goal is approximately 2 pounds per week which represents a net deficit per week of approximately 7000 calories of fat equivalent. This may be achieved by a reduction in caloric intake or through increased exercise and more reasonably a proper combination of both.

Weight loss may be approached through individual effort, group therapy, or a combination of these. Fundamentally, a sound dietary program is one in which the patient receives an adequate level of essential nutrients in a palatable and acceptable form and does not become too hungry. By and large, diets that furnish approximately 1200–1400 calories per day for women and 1400–1600 calories per day for men will enable them to achieve these goals. Diets of less than 1000 calories per day are generally not accepted over a long period of time and often do not contain the proper level of all important nutrients. Such low caloric diets are to be discouraged. Starvation or near total caloric restriction may sometimes be used as a temporary therapeutic measure for grossly overweight patients who have not responded to other methods of treatment. Such programs should not, however, be undertaken without the close supervision of a physician, and the patient should usually be hospitalized. Selected days of fasting, such as one out of every four, provide satisfaction for many individuals and, in general, offer a method of reducing calories, but again the emphasis should be on learning a new life style that is compatible with achieving and maintaining lower weight. A great variety of specialized diets primarily emphasizing high levels of protein have been advocated from time to time. It is true that dietary carbohydrate and also sodium tend to favor the retention of fluids and, hence, obscure fat catabolism and accompanying weight loss as measured by the scale. Over a long period these special type diets do not offer a significant advantage over a properly balanced diet contributing all important nutrients at appropriate levels.

Many drugs have been advocated from time to time in weight reduction programs: desiccated thyroid preparations, a great variety of diuretics, and a variety of amphetamines and related compounds are illustrative of these medications. There is very little evidence to recommend any such preparations in a weight reduction program and certainly some of them, such as the amphetamines, may be dangerous. They are not recommended.

Citrus Fruits for Reducing Diets

Citrus fruits and citrus juices offer a number of advantages in an appropriate diet for weight reduction. Jolliffe emphasized that any good reducing diet should provide at least one serving of citrus each day, most commonly taken at breakfast. A 6-oz. serving of orange juice, for example, provides approximately 80 calories primarily in the form of simple sugars, readily available sources of "energizing" calories. A similar amount of grapefruit juice provides somewhat fewer calories, 72. Many people complain of being hungry on many weight reduction programs, and a serving of citrus functions as an excellent appetite appeaser and again provides a rapidly available form of carbohydrates as an "energizer."

Since citrus products are devoid of fat, no "fat" calories are derived from this concentrated source of energy. Citrus products in the weight reduction diet are both appetite satisfying and taste appealing. For those individuals who appear to be sensitive to the fluid-retaining effects of sodium, it is important to note that citrus products contain practically no sodium and, hence, minimize the undesirable impact of sodium on fluid retention. A sample weight reduction diet plan which provides the daily food and nutrition allowances is presented in the Appendix.

Needs for Calories and Exercise

The primary nutritional requirement is for calories. No diet may be considered adequate unless energy balance is considered, and this becomes particularly important as the caloric intake is reduced, due to weight reduction programs or economic circumstances. It is generally true that as the caloric intake is reduced, it becomes increasingly difficult to provide a well-balanced diet which includes all of the required nutrients in appropriate amounts. We have in this country noted a continued reduction, although modest, in the recommended daily allowances for calories. This in part reflects the increasing sedentary habits of our society. Despite this recommended decrease in daily caloric allowances, obesity and excess weight remain major health problems for Americans and are certainly the most serious nutritional problems. Alcohol all too often represents a major source of calories and a negative impact on nutritional status (138).

Energy needs are related to calories required for:

1. Basal metabolism.
2. Specific dynamic action.
3. Extra heat production for the maintenance of body temperature in a cold environment.
4. A variety of physical activities.
5. Growth, tissue repairs, and the increased calories required for the developing fetus in pregnancy and for the losses of calories during lactation.

Of great significance in estimating caloric requirements is the physiological difference between men and women with respect to caloric need; for example, the RDA of calories for the male aged 23–50 is 2700, while for the female in the same age bracket it is 2000. Pregnancy and lactation increase the recommended caloric allowances for the female by 300 and 500 calories per day, respectively (see Table 3 in Appendix).

Unfortunately, we do not place enough emphasis on the importance of regular exercise, not only in weight reduction programs but in maintaining good muscle tone and strength as well as general good health. Properly structured exercise programs exert a very favorable effect in lowering blood cholesterol, thus reducing risk of atherosclerotic coronary heart disease (139, 140).

A number of very simple, enjoyable, highly beneficial exercises can be introduced into the daily program. For example, walking at the rate of 4 miles per hour will expend calories at the rate of approximately 100 per mile or from 350 to 400 calories per hour. Swimming may expend from 300 to 700 calories per hour, depending upon the intensity of the stroke; skiing utilizes from 600 to 700 calories per hour, and even dancing can result in the expenditure of 200–400 calories per hour. It is evident then that exercise can not only be beneficial but also enjoyable, which it should be. A wide variety of sports provides opportunities for individuals to do their own "thing" in their own way.

A word of caution regarding exercise is important, particularly for individuals over 40 or for those who have or have suspected evidence of cardiovascular disease. Such individuals should be carefully evaluated by their physician and should have a gradually accelerating exercise program developed for them. By all means one should avoid sudden "bursts" of exercise, and a careful warm-up period should be utilized before undertaking any reasonably vigorous exercise. Table 12 in the Appendix lists a wide variety of activities and the approximate energy expenditure for each.

Nutritional Factors for Optimal Performance

A considerable number of nutritional and dietary recommendations have been made from time to time, indicating some unusual benefit to be derived from a given particular diet or spectrum of nutrients. The literature has been reviewed by Consolazio and includes studies conducted by the U.S. Army Medical Research and Nutrition Laboratories (141). In general these studies show that the daily nutrient recommended allowances of the National Research Council are quite liberal for heavy work performance and that there is no demonstrated need for additional nutrient supplements, providing the caloric requirements are met and the calories are provided in a balanced diet with appropriate representation from the various food groups. There is then no sound experimental evidence that has been confirmed in well-controlled studies to suggest that there is a magical nutrient formula that will provide for unusual or unexpected higher physical performance. There is no doubt that athletic coaches and others will continue to search for the "magic" food or nutrient that will result in some startling new high level performance or record. Such an achievement, however, does not permit a cause and effect conclusion without appropriate control studies. This is a most difficult field for experimentation.

This is not to conclude that no evidence is available to support a preferential utilization of certain nutrients in the performance of exercise. For example, the quantity, quality, and character of the calories available for muscular contractions, the level of maximal oxygen uptake, climate conditions, and body hydration are most important determinants for optimal athletic performance. Some data are available that show that the human capacity for prolonged exercise is enhanced after eating a diet rich in carbohydrates. Experimental subjects placed on heavy exercise programs and given a high carbohydrate diet consistently performed better during a prolonged period of heavy exercise than those subjects who were given a "mixed" diet with the initial level of muscle glycogen determining the quality of performance. This study suggests that the prior depletion of glycogen reserves by a very low carbohydrate diet followed by a very high carbohydrate diet for a few days immediately preceding long-term physical exercise results in an accumulation of muscle glycogen which is beneficial to the athlete. Many factors are variable in such studies, and conclusions all too often tend to rely on logic and theory rather than on solid biochemical and metabolic evidence. Certainly it would be helpful to learn whether or not there are certain circumstances under which the body more readily mobilizes and utilizes the adipose tissue reserves for heavy exercise demands. It appears that muscle glycogen reserves are important to muscular performance since as glycogen levels approach low values there is a marked reduction in running speed. One negative factor was noted in the program for increasing muscle glycogen. It appears that glycogen deposition tends to cause water retention in both liver and muscle, resulting in increased body weight which in turn reduces the ability of the human being to take up oxygen maximally (142).

Although one must not conclude from these studies that carbohydrate is the "magic" nutrient, this and other studies certainly suggest that readily available carbohydrate contributes prominently to man's energy needs and is particularly important, and, in fact, critical, for the proper metabolism of tissues of the brain and central nervous system (128). Although the brain and central nervous system represent only a small part of the body, their rate of metabolism is high and has been estimated to use as much as 25 per cent of the energy used in resting metabolism in man. There is little doubt that for the rapid replenishment of circulating blood glucose, the simple sugars of orange juice provide a quick source of energy.

NUTRITIONAL CONSIDERATIONS IN OBSTETRICS AND GYNECOLOGY (143)

Nutritional requirements during the physiological stresses of pregnancy are increased. The RDA reflect these considerations with regard to increased allowances for calories, protein, vitamin A, vitamin E, ascorbic acid, folacin (folic acid), niacin, riboflavin, thiamin, pyridoxine, vitamin B_{12}, and the minerals calcium, phosphorus, zinc, iodine, and magnesium (19). Interestingly, the RDA for iron is the same for the adult or pregnant female and during lactation (18 mg. per day). This is despite the common occurrence of iron deficiency anemia during pregnancy (144). At age 51 and older the RDA for iron drops to 10 mg. per day.

Ascorbic acid obviously plays an important part in growth and development and is abundant in active and growing tissues. These factors are reflected in the increased RDA for ascorbic acid of 60 mg. and 80 mg. per day during pregnancy and lactation, respectively. Since ascorbic acid is not stored and a daily allowance is recommended, orange juice and other citrus products provide ideal sources for meeting the increased requirement. A 6-oz. serving (180 ml.) will provide 80 mg. of ascorbic acid in a readily available, palatable, and inexpensive form. For those individuals preferring a slightly less caloric and less sweet citrus drink, grapefruit juice provides 70 mg. of ascorbic acid in a 6-oz. serving. Both of these levels exceed the RDA of ascorbic acid for the pregnant female. Appropriate selection of citrus products at reasonable serving levels will fulfill the RDA for ascorbic acid during the physiological stress of pregnancy, eliminating the need for synthetic vitamin supplementation at least with respect to ascorbic acid.

Javert of the Woman's Clinic of the New York Hospital has established a treatment regimen for habitual aborters which includes liberal use of orange juice and additional supplements of ascorbic acid and vitamin K, along with an optimal diet in all other respects (145). Decidual hemorrhage is a major factor in spontaneous abortion and this preventive therapy is aimed primarily at minimizing its risk. The rationale for this management program is based on the observation that during the first half of pregnancy, plasma levels of ascorbic acid appear to be lower than desired (average 0.42 mg. per 100 ml. of plasma). Since there appears to be a distinct correlation between decidual hemorrhage and more significant levels of ascorbic acid deficiency, it is thought that decidual hemorrhage may be one manifestation of scurvy. This is theoretically reasonable based on the consideration that the blood vessel integrity is maintained by an intercellular cement substance known to require ascorbic acid for its normal synthesis.

It is interesting that Javert considers orange juice or orange fruit slices as sources of ascorbic acid to be therapeutically superior to synthetic ascorbic acid. Again factors other than ascorbic acid itself present in orange juice may explain this difference since there is no demonstrated chemical difference between the ascorbic acid in citrus and that obtained as a chemical substance. It must be stressed that this observation is only one of many reputed to demonstrate a superior advantage for citrus juice or fruit over synthetic ascorbic acid. One must be cautious regarding these interpretations in view of the complex of nutrients and chemical substances present in citrus or in citrus juices that may have an unappreciated bearing on the observed effects.

A similar study by Murphy (146), on the effectiveness of a nutritionally based treatment program for threatened abortion, indicates that a high intake of citrus fruits and juices as well as ascorbic acid represents important, useful, supportive, and therapeutic measures.

Ascorbic Acid for Menorrhagia

An inadequate tissue level of ascorbic acid is responsible for a breakdown of the mesenchymal tissues, resulting in bleeding even though the blood coagulation system and the platelets are normal. Although all hemostatic tests are normal, the tourniquet test is positive. A positive result in this test along with a lack of ascorbic acid in the blood is associated with scurvy and has been considered by Quick to be the first identified bleeding disease in man (147). There is a tendency in functional menorrhagia toward increased bleeding attributed to increased capillary permeability and fragility (148). Reduction in capillary strength just before menstruation has also been noted, suggesting a transient reduction of ascorbic acid at this particular time possibly associated with an increased metabolic need. A number of studies have reported the usefulness of ascorbic acid, again combined with citrus bioflavonoids, in the treatment of excessive uterine bleeding (149). It is unfortunate that these studies generally utilize a complicated therapeutic regimen which makes it most difficult to evaluate the critical component that may be effective.

Weight Gain and Nutrition during Pregnancy— A New Look (150)

For some years there has been a sustained effort to restrict weight gain during pregnancy. This was based in part on concern over an increased incidence of toxemia of pregnancy often associated with excessive weight gain and fluid retention. Recently, the total, cumulative, extra energy cost of pregnancy has been determined, and it has been found on the average to be "remarkably constant regardless of dietary intake or body build." In general, it was noted that these extra calories during pregnancy are derived from carbohydrate in preference to fat. The additional calories required during pregnancy were determined by the amount of oxygen consumed under carefully controlled and measured conditions. "The total cumulative resting extra caloric expenditure (due to pregnancy) turns out to average 27,120 plus or minus 2,175 kilocalories (kcal) for the ten subjects. The mean daily increase for all subjects tested amounts to just over 100 kcal for the whole period of pregnancy with a median value of nine kcal for the first trimester, 84 kcal for the second and 216 kcal for the third."

Folic Acid Deficiency during Pregnancy (151, 152)

Folacin deficiency is one of the most common of the water-soluble vitamin deficiencies. It is of particular concern for women, who apparently have the ability to develop mild to severe folic acid deficiency in a rather insidious but often accelerating fashion. The classical and characteristic megaloblastic anemia of fulminating folic acid deficiency is not often documented in the American nutritional scene except as a terminal event in the deficiency state. A whole spectrum of events may occur in association with progressive folic acid deficiency, and this same sequence of events from a mild to a florid form of folic acid deficiency may occur during pregnancy (153, 154). Folic acid is not widely distributed in foods, and perhaps more important, cooking, either with high and long exposure to heat or in large volumes of water, may destroy or remove large amounts of what folic acid there is.

Citrus fruits, particularly, orange juice, contain very significant amounts of folic acid, offering an important nutritional advantage for these products in the potential prevention of folic acid deficiency, particularly during pregnancy when the requirements for this vitamin appear to be substantially greater. The RDA for folic acid for the normal adult female is 0.4 mg., but during pregnancy it is 0.8 mg. Considering the availability of folic acid in the general food supply, it may be difficult to achieve this level of intake during pregnancy unless there is careful selection of food.

It has also been shown that folic acid deficiency may be associated with abnormal cervical cytology, that is, the cells of the cervix may undergo abnormal differentiation with atypical morphology. These changes are of clinical importance in the diagnosis of folic acid deficiency and may be of even greater clinical importance in the cytological diagnosis of premalignant cervical lesions, particularly during pregnancy. Primarily, however, cellular dysplasia or other abnormal cytology in pregnancy should certainly suggest the possibility of significant folic acid deficiency.

There is little doubt that megaloblastic anemia developing during pregnancy is highly related to folic acid deficiency (155–58). In addition, thrombocytopenia is not uncommon in patients with megaloblastic anemia. These two factors, then, may relate significantly as complications of folic acid deficiency in pregnancy which may increase the need for transfusion therapy or the hazard of hemorrhage at the time of delivery. These must be considered potential "reproductive complications" of folic acid deficiency, i.e., megaloblastic anemia and thrombocytopenia with secondary hemorrhage with an associated increased risk of transfusion therapy. From the preventive point of view, it is important to insure an adequate dietary level of folic acid throughout pregnancy (159).

Abruptio placentae and folic acid deficiency have been associated by a number of studies. Preliminary results indicate a fivefold greater risk of abruptio placentae in women with folic acid deficiency.

The search for nutritional and other etiological factors in pre-eclampsia and eclampsia continues to be of great interest. All of these studies remain in the doubtful or unproved category; but, as has been true in the clinical evaluation of all nutritional deficiencies, a wide spectrum of problems may be associated. It is most difficult to identify the nutritional deficiency with the disease entity on a cause and effect basis. This has often led to the discredit of nutritional studies and emphasizes the importance of carefully performed and well-controlled clinical investigations in these very important areas.

There is little doubt, however, that folic acid deficiency remains a very common problem in pregnancy and can lead to serious difficulties. Most of these difficulties are preventable through dietary management, regularly utilizing foods that contain and contribute substantial amounts of folic acid.

Folic Acid Deficiency and Oral Contraceptives

Oral contraceptives have become a common medication for women in the United States and many other countries. As might be anticipated, a number of undesirable side effects have been identified with these agents. Recently folic acid deficiency and anemia have been described in association with the use of oral contraceptives (160), and there does appear to be a cause and effect relationship between them. Folic acid deficiency that is associated with the orally administered contraceptive agents does not necessarily imply the discontinuance of the contraceptive drug but does indicate an increased need for folic acid. Folic acid deficiency caused by contraceptive drugs must be considered relatively rare when compared to the usual causes of deficiency associated with malnutrition, malabsorption, alcoholism, and pregnancy.

Folic Acid and the American Diet

Generally, folic acid deficiency of varying severity is common and particularly so during pregnancy. There are four principal causes: inadequate dietary intake, excessive demands by tissues of the body in metabolic derangements such as in pregnancy, inadequate absorption, and metabolic derangements from a variety of causes. Moderate folic acid deficiency is best diagnosed by the evaluation of this vitamin in serum, using microbiological assays, or by the actual hematological response to an appropriate dose of folic acid usually from 50 to 200 μg. per day for 10 days intramuscularly. A daily intake of 50 μg. of crystalline folic acid will prevent depletion of serum folic acid and will probably permit tissue storage. This level, then, is taken as the minimum daily requirement and is not to be confused with the Recommended Daily Allowance (RDA) which is 0.4 mg. for both males and females 11 years of age and older.

Because of the frequency of folic acid deficiency in the general population, and particularly during pregnancy, the question arises as to the adequacy of the "usual" American diet in supplying sufficient folic acid, particularly since this vitamin is readily leached from foods during cooking and is also destroyed by heat.

Certainly, the use of fresh and uncooked vegetables, particularly leafy vegetables, which contain folic acid is to be recommended. Fortunately, it has been demonstrated more recently that orange juice is an unusually good source of folic acid with grapefruit juice containing approximately one-third the amount in orange juice.

Nutrition and Dental Health (161)

The quality of nutrition and dietary practices are just as important in the development and maintenance of oral tissues as in the development and maintenance of other body tissues (162). The condition and functioning of the teeth and periodontal tissues are not only important for the health of the oral cavity, but their state of health implicates all the rest of the body. Cheraskin and Ringsdorf suggest that "there is evidence that the oral cavity ages and dies in parallel with the rest of the organism" (163). The reports of one study indicate that the "life expectancy of 2,116 presumably healthy subjects were [sic] found to be closely related to the number of permanent teeth" (163). These important correlations emphasize the need for oral examination and dental care in total health care delivery. Cheraskin has reported that alveolar bone loss proceeds at a much slower rate in persons practicing good oral hygiene and having efficient carbohydrate metabolism.

Cheraskin has studied the relationship between chronologic age and dental age in terms of ascorbic acid nutriture. He evaluated this problem in 139 subjects and, utilizing the criteria for ascorbic acid standards of the Interdepartmental Committee for Nutrition for National Defense, observed that 17.3 per cent of these individuals displayed suboptimal ascorbic acid status. Using a somewhat higher level to delineate between satisfactory and unsatisfactory ascorbic acid nutriture, it was observed that on this basis more than half (53.5 per cent) of the group had suboptimal plasma ascorbic acid levels. Utilizing the sublingual ascorbic acid test, it was noted that

55 per cent of the subjects displayed marginal to poor ascorbic acid status (164–66). An evaluation of the difference between the dental age and chronological age in this group indicated a large percentage that showed chronological-dental age discrepancies. In substance, it was noted that the lingual ascorbic acid test, suggesting poor ascorbic acid nutriture, indicated a significant correlation between chronologic and dental age. Those individuals with optimal ascorbic acid status, as demonstrated by the lingual ascorbic acid test, showed the highest correlation between chronologic and dental age.

In ascorbic acid deficiency, the lesions of the gingiva are particularly striking (167). The lack of the vitamin primarily affects the ability of the cells of connective tissue origin to elaborate their typical collagen intercellular substance. Further, the odontoblasts which form the dentin in developing teeth are of endodermal origin and are readily affected by the deficiency of ascorbic acid. There is also a rarefaction of the alveolar bone comparable to that seen in the ribs and bones of experimental animals and man. Weakness of the supporting bones, as well as a poor quality of the collagen fibers in the supporting structures, allows for a greater mobility of the teeth and a decreased ability to withstand the mechanical stresses involved in chewing. Although gingival and bone changes have been repeatedly noted in ascorbic acid deficiency and scurvy, there is no clear-cut demonstration of the relationship between scurvy and dental care.

Odontoblasts and ameloblasts require ascorbic acid for the formation of their respective connective tissues, dentin, and enamel. Therefore, ascorbic acid deficiency, pre-natally and during early life when teeth are developing, results in improper development of teeth and supporting bone structure.

Cheraskin has studied alveolar bone loss in 53 dental students, half of whom received 8 oz. of orange juice daily for 1 year while the other half had no citrus intake. The nonsupplemented group lost 0.3 per cent more alveolar bone than did the supplemented group. Extrapolations of the results of the study to persons age 50 yielded a 50 per cent projected alveolar bone loss with the nonsupplemented group, but a loss of only 25 per cent for the orange-juice-supplemented group.

Eight nutrition surveys conducted by the Interdepartmental Committee on Nutrition for National Defense showed that decreased dietary intake of ascorbic acid produced clinical findings of bleeding gums or diffusely swollen and friable gums. An intake of ascorbic acid below 30 mg. per day resulted in an increased incidence of the gingival lesions. Low plasma ascorbic acid levels were also correlated with the gingival lesions.

Because nutritional deficiencies do not directly cause the types of disease which require oral surgical treatment, diet is often overlooked in the total management of the oral surgery patient. Nizel (168) states, "the dentist should look upon the diet as an adjuvant similar to analgesics and antibiotics, which is a means of making the patient more comfortable and of speeding recovery. Some of the prime functions of adequate nutrition are: (1) to speed convalescence; (2) to promote wound healing; and (3) to increase the patient's resistance to infection." Certainly citrus products, including juices, are strongly recommended to supply particularly the ascorbic acid nutriture required. In terms of overall dental health, nutritional recommendations are reasonably straightforward (169, 170). Again, it is best to choose a variety of foods from each of the four basic food groups distributed as well as possible in each of the day's meal allotment. The inclusion of foods that require vigorous chewing as a means to stimulate and exercise the various oral tissues and organs is also important. In view of the role of simple sugars and high carbohydrate foods in the development of dental caries, it is particularly recommended that a minimum of sticky, adherent, high carbohydrate foods with a low rate of clearance from the oral cavity should be consumed (171). It is well to point out that while the carbohydrates in citrus foods are primarily simple sugars they are cleared very rapidly from the oral cavity and pose no significant demonstrated threat in carbohydrate-related dental caries etiology. In the choice of between-meal snacks, fresh fruits, vegetables, and fruit juices are preferred from the standpoint of preserving dental health.

NUTRIENT INTERRELATIONSHIPS AND THE MANAGEMENT OF ANEMIAS

Anemia due to iron deficiency is the most common nutritional deficiency in the United States (172); there are certainly physiologically sensitive groups that are generally considered to be at high risk of iron deficiency: the infant after 6 months of age will commonly demonstrate a high incidence of iron deficiency by 12 months of age unless appropriate steps are taken to provide an adequate intake of iron; women during the menstruating years frequently seem to be unable to accumulate adequate iron stores; and during pregnancy women with inadequate iron stores will be unable to meet the ever increasing fetal demands for iron and maintain their own iron nutriture at satisfactory levels.

Currently, the RDA for iron is 18 mg. per day for women of childbearing age; this should be adequate for the accumulation of iron stores so that additional iron therapy during pregnancy will not be required. However, it is generally quite difficult to achieve this level of iron intake with the ordinary diet. This has led to the recommendation for the fortification of a number of commonly used foods with more iron.

Although the iron content of citrus is not significant, its acidic pH and, more particularly, its generous content of ascorbic acid, very significantly favor iron absorption which is a critical factor in minimizing the hazard of iron deficiency anemia (173). The absorption of iron from foods tagged with radioactive iron was greatly enhanced when these foods were taken with orange juice, grapefruit juice, or crystalline ascorbic acid.

As indicated earlier, megaloblastic anemia may occur in association with scurvy, and this condition responds to a combination of folic and ascorbic acids. Ascorbic acid is a key nutrient in the conversion of folic acid to its active form, tetrahydrofolic acid (see Appendix).

Orange juice provides an interesting "marriage" of key nutrients, i.e., folic acid and ascorbic acid, both of which reduce the risk of developing megaloblastic anemia, and because of the acidic character of citrus fruits and juices and the high levels of ascorbic acid contained in these foods, greatly enhances the absorption and utilization of iron so very important in reducing the risk of hypochromic microcytic iron deficiency anemia (174–79).

EFFECTS OF STRESS ON ASCORBIC ACID METABOLISM IN MAN

It has been recognized for many years that stress, whether through physical trauma, acute or chronic illness, or even adverse emotional impact, produces significant alterations in biochemical and hormonal patterns which exert a profound impact on the individual and may significantly alter nutritional status. New research developments are making it apparent that stress as a general reaction can seriously affect the nutritional health of the individual. This creates then a new and important factor in the appropriate selection of food and nutrients in the care and feeding of the sick and otherwise stressed people. Ascorbic acid requirements of man may be significantly increased as the result of such serious stressful circumstances as burns, severe traumatic injuries, acute infections, and rheumatic diseases. These observations have generally resulted in the recommendation that significantly increased therapeutic levels of ascorbic acid be administered in association with such stressful circumstances. This is not to imply that we have an adequate understanding of the mechanism whereby such therapy may be effective (to be discussed in detail under the megavitamin section).

Selye views stress as a nonspecific type of reaction that can be both the cause and the consequence of malnutrition (180, 181). He suggested the concept of the general adaptation syndrome (GAS) to describe the overall sequence of events occurring during stress. One of the first reactions to stress is the elaboration of additional amounts of ACTH by the anterior pituitary gland which acts upon the adrenal to produce a rapid outpouring of corticosteroids and ascorbic acid from the adrenal cortex. Although the exact fate of the ascorbic acid released during stress is still a matter of experimental study and some controversy, it is thought that stress significantly increases the requirement for ascorbic acid probably at the tissue or cellular level. The exact mechanism remains unclear.

The sequence of events in stress-producing situations is initiated by a great variety of "stressor" agents producing the so-called *alarm reaction*. Selye has expressed this as a generalized "call to arms" of the body's defense mechanisms. If the stressor agent is sufficiently severe or continues long enough, the individual or animal may die during the alarm reaction phase. Survival of the alarm reaction or initial stress stage leads then to what Selye calls the stage of resistance, which is the period of adjustment in which certain physiological and biochemical tolerances develop. Should the stress continue as a result of prolonged exposure to the stressor agent, a third phase develops, which is the stage of exhaustion.

The cortical hormones produced by the adrenal under stress exert two major metabolic functions, one aimed primarily at carbohydrate metabolism, the other at mineral metabolism (182). Selye and others have described various derangements in the ability of the adrenal to secrete these hormones which may lead to what Selye has described as *diseases of adaptation*. These seem to be the result of a faulty adaptive response to the stress or stressor agent. It should be emphasized that the general adaptation syndrome is a nonspecific response that may be generated by a great variety of stressor agents. When stress is superimposed on a nutritional disorder, or in the face of nutritional deficits, the effect, in general, is to make a bad condition worse.

Emotional factors or tension are commonly encountered in everyday living, and they exert important stress, initiating the general adaptation syndrome (183). Even in children, stress may be an important influence on nutritional status, growth rate, and nutrient requirement. This emphasizes the importance of evaluating nutritional status and the interaction of stress on the individual and, of course, highlights the need for a well-balanced diet to maintain the physiological economy in the best state of preparation against the impact of stress (184).

A Particular Role for Ascorbic Acid in Stress

Early studies on the effect of ACTH on the adrenals indicated that large amounts of ascorbic acid were lost from the adrenal cortex and in fact served as a measure of the activity of ACTH and the production of corticosteroids by the adrenal cortex. A great many studies have aimed at proving that treatment with large amounts of ascorbic acid would effectively increase the individual's resistance or adaptation to stress. Increased resistance to stress does not appear to occur unless a significant nutritional ascorbic acid deficiency exists.

This observation, that the stimulation of the adrenal gland by ACTH depleted the adrenals of their ascorbic acid content, along with the earlier observation that wound healing was significantly impaired in ascorbic-acid-deficient animals, has provided the basis for the concept that ascorbic acid in some way must be useful in meeting crisis emergencies and that added strength and resistance would be provided by taking a surplus or excess of ascorbic acid.

A careful study has been conducted in an attempt to identify the basic need for ascorbic acid in preventing scurvy and to determine the amount of dietary ascorbic acid needed to maintain a stable turnover of this vitamin. During the course of this study, events occurred which reintroduced the interrelationship between ascorbic acid and stress. Through the use of radioactive ascorbic acid it was established that the range of utilization of ascorbic acid remained remarkably constant at about 3 per cent of the existing body pool per day. These observations remained quite constant from subject to subject until an event occurred which produced substantial emotional stress for one of the subjects. There was then a sudden change in the utilization of ascorbic acid as determined by measuring the labeled vitamin. The rate of utilization increased two- to threefold during a period of severe emotional stress and returned to normal as soon as the crisis passed. Such an observation conducted under controlled clinical circumstances suggests strongly that at least emotional stress can cause a substantial increase in the rate of catabolism of ascorbic acid as compared to normal (185). This is perhaps too limited an observation from which to draw extensive conclusions regarding the value of ascorbic acid in stress.

Other studies have also suggested the importance of ascorbic acid supplementation for the management of a variety of stress-producing conditions such as infections, drug and antibiotic administration, burns, surgical shock, radiation sickness, heavy physical exertion, and exposure to high or low temperatures.

Increased ascorbic acid is important under the stress of physical exertion because it improves the utilization of oxygen and, hence, increases the efficiency of physical energy expenditure by athletes. Prokop has suggested that the ascorbic acid requirements of athletes may be as high as 500 mg. daily (84). Van Huss (186) endeavored to extend the observations of Prokop and determined the physiological effects of synthetic ascorbic acid and natural ascorbic acid contained in orange juice. He reports that those receiving orange juice showed significantly increased pulse pressure in early recovery after strenuous work. The increased pulse pressure is a measure of the result of lowered systolic and diastolic pressures. The rates of recovery of both pressures following the ingestion of ascorbic acid in the form of orange juice were considerably faster.

Again, it is most difficult to assess studies such as these if for no other reason than the differences between synthetic ascorbic acid and orange juice containing ascorbic acid are two quite different modalities with many differences that were not or could not be evaluated. There is no known chemical difference between synthetic ascorbic acid and that contained in orange juice or other natural products. Whether or not other factors are present in citrus which might augment an effect of ascorbic acid is, of course, of interest. This matter of stress and the related role of ascorbic acid continues to be an enigma and must await further experimental studies to more clearly define the interaction between stress and particularly the level of nutrients and the role of nutritional status in resisting the effects of stress. Any stressor agent is likely to produce different patterns of adaptation and response in different subjects, depending on their individual constitutional makeup. It appears that there is a very important, complex relationship between environment and heredity. It is difficult for genes to produce normally functioning individuals unless the environmental factors are also normal. Here the diet and its impact on nutrition must be viewed as a key environmental factor. The genes provide the capacity to respond to a wide variety of environmental conditions in certain ways.

In looking at the nutritional requirements of man, Williams (25) postulates, seemingly quite appropriately, that no two people are exactly alike and that we are all "abnormal normals." He views this individuality of man as extending to nutritional needs with the potential for wide variations in requirements from person to person. Williams reports work showing that some guinea pigs are able to thrive on 1/32 of the amount of ascorbic acid that others require to maintain health. He suggests further that the human needs for this vitamin may vary as widely and suggests extensive studies on this matter (26).

Williams emphasizes the genetotrophic principle which holds that "the nutritional needs of an organism are determined by the characteristics of the metabolic machinery it has inherited." With this concept in mind, we must suspect the prevalence of nutritional disease in any group of people who are fed uniformly a diet designed for the average number of that group.

This interrelationship between genetic and environmental factors with the individuality that is implied suggests a definition for optimum nutrition which each individual should seek. "*Optimum nutrition* is that which provides all dietary nutrients in respect to kind and amount and in proper state of combination or balance so that the organism may always meet the varied exogenous and endogenous stresses of life, whether in health or disease, with a minimal demand or strain on the body's natural homeostatic protective mechanisms" (3). In general, nutritionists have looked to the RDA as a reasonable guide to achieving the goal of optimal nutrition, although it is recognized that these allowances are not indicated as an individual directive nor, in fact, are they intended to meet all of the potential nutrient needs that may be imposed by a wide variety of physiological circumstances. The concept of individuality of man does raise the interesting question of whether the RDA have a sufficient flexibility or safety valve to satisfy the wide and varied needs of individuals.

Current Controversies

There has developed an interesting and sometimes sparkling controversy among that segment of the scientific world that develops its scientific experience on the traditional or "normal" informational data base that has focused primarily on the study of nutritional deficiency diseases. The science of nutrition has basically been built upon the observations accumulated both from natural and experimental circumstances in which signs or symptoms of abnormality were identified and ultimately shown to be related to some specific nutrient (i.e., ascorbic acid in relation to scurvy, vitamin B_1 [thiamin] in beri-beri, etc.). Following these classical demonstrations that a specific nutrient could be related to a deficiency syndrome on a cause and effect basis, many more sophisticated studies have shown that the nutrient in question exerted a specific biochemical function at the enzymatic and cellular levels. Further refinements of the nutritional approach have been associated with attempts to develop latent ("subclinical") deficiencies by examining the nutrient levels in blood, urine, and other available biological tissues. Thus, there has been developed the technology for nutritional evaluation and estimation of nutritional status. Once levels of nutrients have been identified in so-called normal healthy individuals who were consuming the prevailing "normal diet," a basis was established for comparing the normal group with those individuals who exhibited lesser nutrient values of varying degree but without overt manifestations of a deficiency disease. For example, serum levels of ascorbic

77

acid may be very low or even zero in individuals without clinical evidence of scurvy. This kind of observation has created many debates in the scientific literature regarding the adequacy of nutrition based on these still rather crude parameters of measurement. A further sophistication of nutritional evaluation has been developed by demonstrating that certain enzyme activities related to specific nutrients may be deficient at the cellular level, which adds further refinement and scientific evidence for nutritional inadequacy without overt deficiency being demonstrated. Along with these observations has been a very extensive development of food technology in which much has been learned concerning the nutrient content of almost the total spectrum of available foods. A compilation of such data has been made by the U.S. Department of Agriculture and published in Handbook 8.

One question arises. Is there such a thing as "supernutrition"? From the standpoint of nutritional evaluation studies using all of the techniques indicated above, such as nutrient levels in biological tissues of all kinds, the measurement of enzyme activity, and nutritional history, one cannot identify supernutrient levels or supernutritional status. This does not imply, however, that wide ranges of normal levels of tissue nutrients do not exist; in fact, there is increasing evidence that nutritional requirements are highly individualistic.

In essence, then, if we utilize the normal range of tissue nutrients as a basic measure of nutritional adequacy, it is difficult to demonstrate a supernutritional status that might be achieved by taking more nutrients. For example, continued large doses of ascorbic acid maintain serum ascorbic acid at or about a level of 1.5 mg. per cent, but at this level, the renal threshold for the retention of this vitamin is generally exceeded and the excess is excreted in the urine. In other words, there appears to be a natural, built in mechanism, primarily that of excretion via the kidney, which clearly places an upper limit on the circulating serum levels for at least the water-soluble vitamins. With regard to the fat-soluble vitamins, an entirely different situation prevails in which excessive accumulation of tissue vitamins A and D may occur with large dosage levels which have been fairly well defined. Physicians and the public are both cautioned against the excessive utilization of these particular vitamins (187). Ascorbic acid apparently does not pose a significant health hazard even when taken in large doses. Much more study is required, however, to establish the long-term safety of megavitamin doses. Caution is advised. Oxalic acid, one of the end products in the metabolism of ascorbic acid, is excreted in the urine and certain individuals are prone to develop renal calculi. Oxalic acid is regarded as one of the prime "stone formers."

How has the "megavitamin" philosophy developed? The concept that very large doses of nutrients, such as vitamin C, provide special benefits had its great impetus with the publication of the book *Vitamin C and the Common Cold* by Linus Pauling (9). The claims in this book certainly startled the nutritional world and gave rise to much criticism primarily because of the limited evidence upon which Dr. Pauling seemed to have based his conclusions. Subsequently, Dr. Pauling clarified his position in which he specified that "the regular ingestion of 1000 mg. of ascorbic acid leads to the decreased incidence of colds by about 45% and to a decrease in total illness by about 60%." Unfortunately, the ensuing debates between the traditional nutritionists and the "megavitamin" proponents have created more heat than light. More recently Anderson, Reid, and Beaton (188) conducted a careful double-blind trial to test the claim that the intake of 1 gm. of ascorbic acid per day could substantially reduce the frequency and duration of colds. This was a well-planned study with an appropriate placebo group used as a control. In terms of the average number of colds and days of sickness per subject the vitamin group experienced less illness than the placebo group, but the differences were smaller than have been claimed and were not statistically significant. However, there was a statistically significant difference (p less than 0.05) between the two groups in the number of subjects who remained free of illness throughout the study period. Furthermore, the subjects receiving the ascorbic acid experienced approximately 30 per cent fewer days of total disability (confined to the house or off work) than those receiving the placebo, and this difference was statistically highly significant (p less than 0.001). This evidently related to the much lower incidence of constitutional symptoms such as chills and severe malaise (187–91).

What is the conceptual basis upon which these huge pharmocological-type doses of nutrients is advocated? Linus Pauling in 1968 proposed the concept of orthomolecular medicine. "Orthomolecular medicine is the preservation of good health and the treatment of disease by varying the concentrations in the human body of substances that are normally present in the body and are required for health." He further stated, "to achieve the best of health, the rate of intake of essential foods should be such as to establish and maintain the optimum concentration of essential molecules, such as those of ascorbic acid." In this context *ascorbic acid is considered an essential food* required by human beings for life and good health.

Pauling evidently believes that megavitamin therapy is one aspect of orthomolecular medicine and postulates that with time and experience it will be demonstrated that many diseases may be controlled by this form of treatment. For example, there is evidence that schizophrenic patients benefit from treatment with large doses of nicotinic acid in amounts of from 3 to 18 gm. per day along with 3 gm. of ascorbic acid (192). The use of from 400 to 800 mg. of pyridoxine has also been advocated in addition to the above regimen. With regard to vitamins the orthomolecular concept rather reasonably postulates that since metabolic reactions at the molecular and cellular levels are mediated through enzymes and since the coenzyme component of many of these enzymes is derived from vitamins, the huge orthomolecular dose may favorably influence enzyme activity possibly by mass action impact. In certain genetic diseases in which the enzyme is not absent but is present only with greatly diminished activity, it is thought that huge doses of the vitamin with subsequent increased cellular or molecular exposure to high nutrient levels might result ultimately in a more nearly normal level of an "active enzyme." In short, the abnormal component would, in a sense, be overwhelmed by the nutrient supply. All of this is highly speculative and must await extensive well-controlled trials if there is to be any reasonable evidence to support the hypothesis.

Pauling cites as an example of this philosophy the disease methylmalonic aciduria in which there is a deficiency in the activity of the enzyme that catalyzes the conversion of methyl malonic acid to succinic acid. Vitamin B_{12} serves as the coenzyme for this reaction, and the administration of very large doses of vitamin B_{12} may result in an improvement of the conversion reaction to a normal rate for many patients. There is also the question of whether or not huge doses of pyridoxine, shown to be effective in the treatment of pyridoxine-dependent iron deficiency anemia, may function in a similar manner. There is also noted the benefit of huge doses of vitamin D in vitamin D resistant rickets.

No clear-cut conclusions can be drawn at this time regarding the advantages (or possible disadvantages) of the orthomolecular vitamin approach. However, there is little doubt that it has created a substantial new interest in the field of vitamins as potential pharmacological agents over and above their role as "ordinary nutrients." Undoubtedly, a great deal of clinical investigative work will be stimulated by the concept. It may well turn out that the traditional approach to nutrition and the orthomolecular approach may both be right with the two proponents looking at different sides of the same coin.

"NATURAL" FOODS VS. SYNTHETIC FOODS AND NUTRIENTS

Man as a creative and innovative creature is continually attempting to improvise in order to improve on nature. This tendency is particularly great when a strong profit motive adds impetus to creativity. At one time or another man attempts to imitate or duplicate everything good in nature, particularly foods.

With respect to orange juice, many attempts have been made to imitate nature's blend of natural nutrients. Based on the objective data of consumer acceptance one must judge these attempts as only modestly successful despite the tremendous advertising pressure that has been utilized to sway consumer preference.

Looking at it objectively, all too often the synthetic food product focuses on one or two of the nutrients of orange juice, such as ascorbic acid, and attempts to enter into a general competition which essentially says "mine has more than yours." Such goals make little sense in the overall objective of sound food and nutritional practices, and this is recognized in the newly developed federal regulation regarding such practices. One question that arises basic to this problem, is whether or not man can successfully create a mixture of chemicals that exactly duplicates a natural product such as orange juice. When one examines the almost overwhelming array of nutritional and flavorful substances present in natural orange juice, one must question whether or not duplication is a reasonable or practical possibility. It appears that the chemist may simulate but not imitate. The all too frequent emphasis on a specific nutrient in a synthetic product without full attention to the total spectrum of nutrients present in the natural product has little benefit from the nutritional point of view. It is obviously easy to put ascorbic acid into a synthetic orange drink at almost any legally acceptable level, but when one considers, for example, such an important factor as the potassium-sodium ratio in the synthetic product as compared to pure orange juice there are obvious significant differences: the synthetic product invariably has a much higher content of sodium and a lower content of potassium. This is obviously important when one wishes to utilize a product in diets in which sodium or potassium levels are important.

On the other hand, the over-vigorous proponents of the "pure food" run aground on the shoals of poor science when they continue to insist that "the food" is superior to any specific nutrient that may be provided as a synthetic chemical. For example, many studies have been published purporting to demonstrate that orange juice or citrus fruits provide a significant advantage over the chemical substance ascorbic acid. As indicated earlier most of these studies fail to take into consideration that this is a comparison, which, on objective scientific grounds, is impossible, particularly in view of the substantial difficulty of completely imitating a food with chemical mixtures.

There is a lack of sound scientific and valid medical evidence to support the numerous claims for superiority of natural food products in comparison with specific nutrients in a great variety of physiological and disease conditions. It is evident, therefore, that individuals select orange juice for reasons over and above the value contributed by any specific nutrient in it. There is also an increasing concern among the public and among many scientists that synthetic chemicals contained in synthetic food may contain substances whose potential toxicity may become evident only after long years of usage. Although this is an ultraconservative position, it is, nevertheless, one that is of concern to many.

There is a continuing need to educate and advise the health professions and the public regarding the nutrient content of citrus products and their usefulness as a basic component of a well-balanced diet.

One aspect of synthetic versus natural foods is the fact that food, whether a single item or a prepared mixture, provides an important psychodietetic advantage which does not seem to be generally appreciated. This psychodietetic philosophy emphasizes not only nutritional quality but other characteristics important to foods such as their appearance, their appetizing aroma, their subtle or stimulating tastes, and, in fact, the plain pleasurableness of eating. One reflection of this psychodietetic point of view is the tremendous success of cookbooks. In fact, cookbooks have almost become a fad, and there is a cookbook for almost every area of food preparation. One certainly wonders what a poor life we would have if all foods were judged solely on nutritional merit without regard to the fine art of eating and enjoying food which has become such an important part of our culture.

Ruth Leverton, a prominent nutritionist, has summed it up very well by stating, "It is true that the body's requirements for nutritional well being are for nutrients rather than for individual foods per se. Foods however are our best source of nutrients. Not only do foods supply energy, but they supply other factors important to well being, some of which may not have yet been discovered or isolated. The nutrients and energy in food and their interrelationships probably contribute more to the body's well being than the nutrients supplied singly and in chemically purified or synthesized form. Also foods should taste and look good. The search must move full speed ahead however and certainly faster than it has in the past if we are to increase the research base essential for the substantiation for the superiority of foods over simple chemical nutrients" (Nutrition Reviews). In summary, then, a food is much more than just a sum of its individual chemical nutrients.

Nature does a remarkably fine job of producing a uniform orange juice. During 1973 and 1974, samples of frozen concentrated orange juice were collected at regular intervals from twenty-three manufacturers in Florida. Selected nutrients as specified in the Nutrition Labeling Regulations of the United States Food and Drug Administration were analyzed to ascertain their mean concentrations and range and to determine the levels in per cent United States Recommended Daily Allowances of each nutrient in a 6 fluid ounce serving of the properly reconstituted juice. The nutrients analyzed included provitamin A, ascorbic acid, thiamin, riboflavin, niacin, calcium, iron, vitamin B_6, folic acid, phosphorus, magnesium, zinc, copper, and pantothenic acid (193).

The per cent of U.S.-Recommended Dietary Allowances (USRDA) of each nutrient in a serving in this study is shown in Table 3.

These data indicate that the variations of most nutrients in FCOJ are not large. Some of the trace nutrients which are to be declared at the 2 or 4 per cent USRDA per serving levels all averaged higher

than the declared amounts. Also, the FDA Nutrition Labeling Regulations would permit the actual content to be 80 per cent of the
declared amount for the naturally occurring nutrients. For the major
nutrients, i.e., vitamin C, thiamin, and folic acid, for which orange
juice can be considered a significant source, frequent monitoring
may be desirable. The vitamin C level in oranges decreases as the

TABLE 3. MEAN NUTRIENT CONTENTS AND RANGE OF VALUES OF INDIVIDUAL
SAMPLES OF FROZEN CONCENTRATED ORANGE JUICE (FCOJ)
COLLECTED IN 1973 AND 1974

| | | USRDA per serving[1] | |
Nutrient	No. of samples	Range (%)	Mean (%)
Vitamin A	40	0.8– 4.8	1.4
Vitamin C	426	86– 179	131
Thiamin, microbiological	461	7.5–16.3	11.6
Thiamin, thiochrome (AOAC)	298	7.5–12.5	9.8
Riboflavin	100	1.6– 3.5	2.4
Niacin	458	1.5– 2.7	2.0
Calcium	480	0.6– 3.7	1.8
Iron	457	0.2– 4.9	1.1
Vitamin B$_6$	215	3.8– 5.8	4.9
Folic acid Lab. 1	381	8.5–32.5	20.3
Folic acid Lab. 2	216	16.4–26.2	20.3
Phosphorus	326	1.0–12.7	3.3
Magnesium	473	1.5– 7.2	4.9
Zinc	471	0.4– 1.9	0.7
Copper	474	2.5–14.0	4.4
Pantothenic acid	152	2.9– 4.0	3.3

1. Six fl. oz. of reconstituted 12.8° Brix juice.

fruits mature. Thiamin and folic acid, however, were low in samples taken in early season and should also be checked occasionally
during that period.

SUMMARY

This review of the health-related literature has attempted to identify
and emphasize an important new perspective developing in
medicine. The emphasis is on prevention: the new wave of the
future in medicine will be, or certainly should be, disease prevention, especially those chronic and debilitating diseases that have
so far limited our progress in providing and maintaining good health,
particularly in advancing years. In view of the fact that food and

nutrition represent one of the most important continuing environments, an emphasis on nutrition and the application of nutritional knowledge to health should be a new point of emphasis.

The citrus industry continues to advance in the technological improvement of its products with regard to nutritional quality, palatability, and economy. The credibility of its scientific research, its food technological improvements, and its professional and public health education programs may well be measured in part by the ever increasing consumer acceptability and endorsement of its products.

It should not be implied that continuing research and further improvement are not important. With every expansion of knowledge there exists an expanded horizon of things to learn in the future. The Florida Department of Citrus remains dedicated to public nutrition and health both in its educational and in its product improvement programs.

Appendix

THE FLORIDA DEPARTMENT OF CITRUS

The Department of Citrus, a branch of Florida's state government, is the result of legislative acts beginning in 1935 designed to give direction to the growing industry. Since that year, the industry has developed prime fruit and citrus products through the efforts of this cohesive, quality-conscious organization.

The primary concerns of the Florida Department of Citrus include marketing, advertising, merchandising, and regulation of Florida citrus, with deep interest also in the conduct of scientific, market, and economic research.

The Department of Citrus is governed by a board known as the Florida Citrus Commission. The commission consists of twelve industry representatives appointed by the governor of the state for terms of three years each. Four of the members are named each year. All commissioners must have been active in the citrus industry for at least five years prior to appointment. Experience in the growing of citrus, the shipping of fresh citrus, and the processing of citrus products is reflected in the backgrounds of the commission members.

Funds for the operation of the Florida Department of Citrus are obtained through an excise tax placed on each box of citrus fruit moved in commercial channels. Most of the funds are used for advertising and promotional activities.

Possibly the most notable accomplishment of the Department's scientific research program has been the development of the present process for the production of frozen concentrated citrus juices.

Among the activities engaged in by the Florida Department of Citrus are:

1. Supervision of professional advertising campaigns to promote Florida citrus products in the United States, Canada, and abroad.

2. Creation of promotional and merchandising techniques to increase the demand for Florida citrus.

3. Promotion of citrus through an extensive food publicity program that places recipes involving Florida citrus in food publications across the nation.

4. Educational programs that inform health and nutritional leaders of the benefits of Florida citrus to grooming and physical fitness.

5. Publication of visual aids materials and nutritional and grooming publications.

6. Institutional and school marketing programs to instruct those concerned about the nutritional benefits of Florida citrus in school lunch programs, hospital diets, and other related institutional areas.

7. Administration of the Florida Citrus Code which regulates the packing, processing, labeling, and handling of citrus fruits and products and improving these processes and the packaging and quality of citrus fruits and products.

8. Conducting of extensive programs in scientific research to improve upon methods of harvesting and extension of shelf-life of fresh fruit, improvement of fruit and product quality, and the discovery of new uses for Florida citrus.

9. Seeking solutions to economic problems through an economic research program which places emphasis upon studies ranging from consumer preferences to supply management.

10. Protection of both the citrus industry and citrus consumer through adoption of regulations to insure prompt and efficient inspection and proper classification of grades for all citrus moved commercially.

The end results of these efforts are manifest in the continued acceptance and utilization of citrus products by the widest possible spectrum of the consuming public and the ever increasing production of citrus products at a continuing economical cost to meet the ever growing demand.

TABLE 1. Common Laboratory Tests
in Nutritional Disorders

1. Complete urinalysis
2. CBC—blood indices
3. Stool (blood, "fat," parasites)
4. Blood sugar; BUN; creatinine
5. Serum lipids
    Cholesterol (free and esterified)
    Triglycerides
6. Serum proteins (A / G ratio), electrophoretic pattern
7. Liver function pattern (BSP excretion, flocculation tests)
8. Nutrient absorption studies
    Lipid
    Xylose
    Vitamin A tolerance
9. Serum electrolytes; blood pH
10. Calcium, phosphorus, iron

Source: Krehl (12).

TABLE 2. Some Special Nutrient
Measurements

1. Serum vitamin A and carotene
2. Urinary thiamin and riboflavin excretion
3. Pyridoxine nutriture—tryptophan load test
4. Folic acid serum level
5. Vitamin B_{12} serum level
6. Ascorbic acid in plasma vs. ascorbic acid in WBC layer
7. Vitamin E—RBC hemolysis and serum vitamin E levels

Source: Krehl (12).

TABLE 3. Food and Nutrition Board, National Academy of Sciences–National Research Council Recommended Daily Dietary Allowances (Revised 1974)[1]

(Designed for the maintenance of good nutrition of practically all healthy people in the U.S.A.)

	Weight (kg.)	Weight (lbs.)	Height (cm.)	Height (in.)	Energy (kcal.)[2]	Protein (gm.)	Vitamin A activity (RE)[3]	Vitamin A activity (IU)	Vitamin D activity (IU)	Vitamin E activity[5] (IU)	Ascorbic acid (mg.)	Folacin[6] (mg.)	Niacin[7] (µg.)	Riboflavin (mg.)	Thiamin (mg.)	Vitamin B6 (mg.)	Vitamin B12 (µg.)	Calcium (mg.)	Phosphorus (mg.)	Iodine (µg.)	Iron (mg.)	Magnesium (mg.)	Zinc (mg.)
Infants 0.0–0.5	6	14	60	24	kg. × 117	kg. × 2.2	420[4]	1,400	400	4	35	50	5	0.4	0.3	0.3	0.3	360	240	35	10	60	3
0.5–1.0	9	20	71	28	kg. × 108	kg. × 2.0	400	2,000	400	5	35	50	8	0.6	0.5	0.4	0.3	540	400	45	15	70	5
Children 1–3	13	28	86	34	1,300	23	400	2,000	400	7	40	100	9	0.8	0.7	0.6	1.0	800	800	60	15	150	10
4–6	20	44	110	44	1,800	30	500	2,500	400	9	40	200	12	1.1	0.9	0.9	1.5	800	800	80	10	200	10
7–10	30	66	135	54	2,400	36	700	3,300	400	10	40	300	16	1.2	1.2	1.2	2.0	800	800	110	10	250	10
Males 11–14	44	97	158	63	2,800	44	1,000	5,000	400	12	45	400	18	1.5	1.4	1.6	3.0	1,200	1,200	130	18	350	15
15–18	61	134	172	69	3,000	54	1,000	5,000	400	15	45	400	20	1.8	1.5	2.0	3.0	1,200	1,200	150	18	400	15
19–22	67	147	172	69	3,000	54	1,000	5,000	400	15	45	400	20	1.8	1.5	2.0	3.0	800	800	140	10	350	15
23–50	70	154	172	69	2,700	56	1,000	5,000		15	45	400	18	1.6	1.4	2.0	3.0	800	800	130	10	350	15
51+	70	154	172	69	2,400	56	1,000	5,000		15	45	400	16	1.5	1.2	2.0	3.0	800	800	110	10	350	15
Females 11–14	44	97	155	62	2,400	44	800	4,000	400	12	45	400	16	1.3	1.2	1.6	3.0	1,200	1,200	115	18	300	15
15–18	54	119	162	65	2,100	48	800	4,000	400	12	45	400	14	1.4	1.1	2.0	3.0	1,200	1,200	115	18	300	15
19–22	58	128	162	65	2,100	46	800	4,000	400	12	45	400	14	1.4	1.1	2.0	3.0	800	800	100	18	300	15
23–50	58	128	162	65	2,000	46	800	4,000		12	45	400	13	1.2	1.0	2.0	3.0	800	800	100	18	300	15
51+	58	128	162	65	1,800	46	800	4,000		12	45	400	12	1.1	1.0	2.0	3.0	800	800	80	10	300	15
Pregnant					+300	+30	1,000	5,000	400	15	60	800	+2	+0.3	+0.3	2.5	4.0	1,200	1,200	125	18+[8]	450	20
Lactating					+500	+20	1,200	6,000	400	15	80	600	+4	+0.5	+0.3	2.5	4.0	1,200	1,200	150	18	450	25

1. The allowances are intended to provide for individual variations among most normal persons as they live in the United States under usual environmental stresses. Diets should be based on a variety of common foods in order to provide other nutrients for which human requirements have been less well defined. See text for more detailed discussion of allowances.

2. Kilojoules (kJ.) = 4.2 × kcal.

3. Retinol equivalents.

4. Assumed to be all as retinol in milk during the first six months of life. All subsequent intakes are assumed to be half as retinol and half as β-carotene when calculated from international units. As retinol equivalents, three-fourths are as retinol and one-fourth as β-carotene.

5. Total vitamin E activity, estimated to be 80 per cent as α-tocopherol and 20 per cent other tocopherols.

6. The folacin allowances refer to dietary sources as determined by Lactobacillus casei assay. Pure forms of folacin may be effective in doses less than one-fourth of the recommended dietary allowance.

7. Although allowances are expressed as niacin, it is recognized that on the average 1 mg. of niacin is derived from each 60 mg. of dietary tryptophan.

8. This increased requirement cannot be met by ordinary diets; therefore, the use of supplemental iron is recommended.

TABLE 4. CERTIFIED CITRUS FRUIT FOR USE AT CANNING
AND CONCENTRATING PLANTS

(By Seasons: August 1–July 31. In terms of 1 3/5 bushel boxes.)

Season	Grapefruit	Oranges	Tangerines	Other[1]	Total
1959–1960[2]	14,297,801	70,133,784	540,505	79,157	85,051,247
1960–1961[3]	15,712,884	69,500,267	1,588,158	13,657	86,814,966
1961–1962	16,631,332	91,808,094	1,235,373	22,919	109,697,718
1962–1963[4]	16,133,940	62,725,790	400,032	13,958	79,273,720
1963–1964[5]	11,817,312	45,385,461	1,132,849	35,271	58,370,893
1964–1965[6]	16,283,174	69,648,568	1,169,255	18,374	87,119,371
1965–1966	20,027,810	82,972,305	869,488	11,780	103,881,383
1966–1967	26,697,665	124,250,589	1,067,510	25,580	152,041,344
1967–1968	18,557,423	85,514,981	665,907	315,712	105,054,023
1968–1969[7]	26,267,992	120,207,786	1,073,001	593,083	148,141,862
1969–1970	23,329,125	128,577,603	617,535	810,287	153,334,550
1970–1971[8]	28,030,250	132,743,158	1,038,557	909,134	162,721,099
1971–1972	30,031,212	130,646,685	1,853,944	844,755	163,376,596
1972–1973	28,336,558	158,829,153	1,329,267	1,269,111	189,764,089
1973–1974	29,425,512	162,995,467	1,484,086	1,185,485	195,090,550

SOURCE: Division of Fruit and Vegetable Inspection, Florida Department of Agriculture and Consumer Services, Winter Haven, Florida.
1. Includes Clementines, King Orange, Satsumas, Sour Oranges, Page, Lee, Osceola, limes, lemons, Ponkans, Gronges, and K-Early.
2. Includes 430 boxes oranges imported from Cuba.
3. Includes 100,522 boxes oranges imported from Cuba and 81 boxes grapefruit and 75,233 boxes oranges from Texas.
4. Includes 1,705 boxes grapefruit and 62,301 boxes oranges imported from Mexico, and 67 boxes grapefruit and 745 boxes oranges imported from Haiti.
5. Includes 312,454 boxes of oranges imported from Puerto Rico, Haiti, Mexico, or the Dominican Republic.
6. Includes 3,803 boxes of oranges imported from Haiti.
7. Includes 82,902 boxes of oranges from Texas.
8. Includes 534 boxes of grapefruit and 45,274 boxes of oranges from Texas.

TABLE 5. Florida Production of Citrus Concentrate 1973–74

Size		Frozen orange	Frozen grapefruit		Frozen blend	Frozen tangerine
46/6 oz. (includes 48/8 oz.)	SA[1] US[2]	242,825 22,967,000			136,782	108,087
24/6 oz.	SA US		SA US	8,545 1,353,561		
24/12 oz.	SA US	161,098 23,941,397	SA US	— 272,049		
24/16 oz.	SA US	35,768 7,512,635				
12/32 oz.		3,080,566	SA US	— 181,723		
Other sizes converted to 12/32 oz.		1,787,964				
Total cases all sizes		59,729,253		1,815,878	136,782	108,087
Total sizes converted to gallons		143,703,506		2,689,638	153,881	121,602
Bulk gals.		111,689,164		9,335,289	5,429	1,026,425
Gross gals.		255,392,670		12,024,927	159,310	1,148,027
Less reprocessed gals.		83,546,774		2,999,026	148,298	128,770
Net gals.		171,845,896		9,025,901	11,012	1,019,257

Source: Florida Canners Association, Winter Haven, Florida.
1. SA = sweetener added.
2. US = unsweetened.

TABLE 6. Processed Concentrated Orange Juice, Frozen
Concentrated Orange Juice, and Frozen Grapefruit
Annual Packs in Florida, Seasons of
1945–46 to 1973–74, Inclusive

Year	Processed concentrated orange juice (gals.)	Frozen concentrated orange juice (gals.)	Frozen grapefruit concentrate (gals.)
1945–46	244,000	226,000	
1946–47	1,447,000	559,000	
1947–48	1,739,000	1,935,000	
1948–49	1,897,000	10,232,000	116,123
1949–50	1,529,422	21,647,447	1,584,561
1950–51	2,529,671	30,757,656	187,903
1951–52	1,897,848	44,030,633	1,097,564
1952–53	536,660	46,553,695	1,226,485
1953–54	1,339,222	65,531,204	1,656,469
1954–55	1,531,449	64,685,956	1,155,314
1955–56	1,085,697	70,224,053	2,511,831
1956–57	1,801,283	72,011,741	2,949,072
1957–58	1,149,081	57,150,566	3,330,301
1958–59	547,280	79,910,670	4,952,488
1959–60	377,877	78,149,306	1,613,462
1960–61	154,911	84,298,114	3,841,462
1961–62	277,501	116,081,547	3,162,798
1962–63	54,360	51,647,737	2,323,381
1963–64	41,108	53,674,426	2,572,661
1964–65	69,763	88,868,804	3,999,657
1965–66	48,506	70,831,316	3,970,546
1966–67	119,027	127,610,559	5,484,816
1967–68	22,374	83,697,047	1,813,964
1968–69	31,126	103,731,616	5,917,390
1969–70	34,293	124,947,460	4,293,843
1970–71	27,830	125,173,952	6,876,309
1971–72		134,170,848	8,797,516
1972–73		176,073,382	8,657,624
1973–74		171,845,896	9,025,901

Source: Florida Canners Association, Winter Haven, Florida.

TABLE 7. CONCENTRATED PROCESSED GRAPEFRUIT, FROZEN BLENDED
CONCENTRATE, AND FROZEN TANGERINE CONCENTRATE
SEASONS OF 1953–54 TO 1973–74, INCLUSIVE

Year	Processed grapefruit (gal.)	Frozen blend (gal.)	Processed blend and tangerine (gal.)	Frozen tangerine (gal.)
1953–54	55,372	965,430		443,105
1954–55	31,860	560,545		877,011
1955–56	30,719	954,142	25,055	618,986
1956–57	59,105	596,731	32,431	792,516
1957–58	107,896	506,915		146,576
1958–59	165,115	689,521	188,154	1,151,782
1959–60	27,390	284,276		319,671
1960–61	19,947	255,584	21,285	1,406,694
1961–62	116,171	266,598	3,989	1,370,187
1962–63	36,340	53,242	20,821	204,458
1963–64	21,375	130,430		1,145,495
1964–65	54,946	69,599		1,153,569
1965–66	30,539	50,487		715,490
1966–67	32,011	29,099		1,119,869
1967–68		10,349		581,966
1968–69	38,742	36,310		1,050,946
1969–70	39,752	16,285		785,150
1970–71	89,004	17,913		1,089,882
1971–72	31,282	22,002		1,219,793
1972–73		3,478		1,072,201
1973–74		11,012		1,019,257

Number of field boxes of grapefruit used for canning frozen grapefruit, processed
grapefruit, and frozen blend for the 1973–74 season: 8,731,963
Number of field boxes of oranges used for canning frozen orange concentrate,
processed orange, and frozen blend for the 1973–74 season: 132,475,347
Number of field boxes of tangerines used for canning frozen tangerine concentrate
for the 1973–74 season: 879,422

SOURCE: Florida Canners Association, Winter Haven, Florida.

TABLE 8. Effect of Different Storage Times and Temperatures
and of Boiling on Ascorbic Acid in
Freshly Squeezed Orange Juice

Treatment	Total[1]	L-AscA[2]	DHA[3]	DKA[4]	TAV[5]	Change (%)
		(mg. per 100 gm.)				
Freshly squeezed	38.50	36.33	0.07	2.11	36.40	
Refrigerated 24 hours	38.75	35.26	1.43	2.06	36.69	+0.79
48 hours	39.20	35.60	1.43	2.06	37.17	+2.11
72 hours	39.50	35.20	1.94	2.46	37.14	+2.03
1 week	37.25	33.08	1.83	2.34	34.91	−4.09
Held at room temperature 24 hours	38.25	35.43	0.75	2.07	36.18	−0.60
48 hours	36.50	33.96	0.90	1.66	34.86	−4.23
72 hours	40.25	37.01	1.07	2.17	38.08	+4.61
1 week	38.35	34.93	3.42	1.17	36.10	−0.82
Boiled	34.75	32.55	1.61	0.59	34.16	−6.15

Source: Lopez, Krehl, and Good (37).
1. Total-total osazone-yielding material.
2. L-AscA-L-ascorbic acid.
3. DHA-dehydroascorbic acid.
4. DKA-2,3 diketogulonic acid.
5. TAV-total active vitamin (L-AscA + DHA).

TABLE 9. Effect of Different Storage Times and Temperatures
and of Boiling on Ascorbic Acid in an
Ascorbic Acid Solution

Treatment	Total[1]	L-AscA[2]	DHA[3]	DKA[4]	TAV[5]	Change (%)
		(mg. per 100 gm.)				
Freshly prepared	52.32	51.06	1.05	0.21	52.11	
Refrigerated 24 hours	49.87	43.92	5.40	0.55	49.32	− 5.35
48 hours	51.76	44.08	6.81	0.87	50.89	− 2.34
72 hours	48.42	37.87	8.65	1.90	46.52	−10.72
1 week	48.09	26.77	15.95	5.37	42.72	−18.01
Held at room temperature 24 hours	48.07	36.59	9.77	2.71	46.36	−11.03
48 hours	46.60	28.54	11.97	6.27	40.33	−22.60
72 hours	44.85	21.48	12.37	11.00	33.85	−35.04
1 week	41.51	7.11	10.90	23.50	18.01	−65.43
Boiled	45.95	39.62	5.27	1.06	44.89	−13.85

Source: Lopez, Krehl, and Good (37).
1. Total-total osazone-yielding material.
2. L-AscA-L-ascorbic acid.
3. DHA-dehydroascorbic acid.
4. DKA-2,3 diketogulonic acid.
5. TAV-total active vitamin (L-AscA + DHA).

TABLE 10. COMPOSITION OF FOODS, 100 GRAMS, EDIBLE PORTION

Food and description	Water (%)	Food energy (cals.)	Protein (gm.)	Fat (gm.)	Carbohydrate Total (gm.)	Carbohydrate Fiber (gm.)	Ash (gm.)	Calcium (mg.)	Phosphorus (mg.)	Iron (mg.)	Sodium (mg.)	Potassium (mg.)	Vitamin A value (I.U.)	Thiamin (mg.)	Riboflavin (mg.)	Niacin (mg.)	Ascorbic acid (mg.)
Oranges, raw																	
Peeled fruit																	
All commercial varieties	86.0	49	1.0	.2	12.2	.5	.6	41	20	.4	1	200	200	.10	.04	.4	(50)
California																	
Navels (winter oranges)	85.4	51	1.3	.1	12.7	.5	.5	40	22	.4	1	194	(200)	.10	.04	.4	(61)
Valencias (summer oranges)	85.6	51	1.2	.3	12.4	(.5)	.5	40	22	.8	1	190	(200)	.10	.04	.4	(49)
Florida																	
All commercial varieties	86.4	47	.7	(.2)	12.0	(.5)	.7	43	17	.2	1	(206)	(200)	.10	.04	.4	(45)
Fruit, including peel (California Valencias)	82.3	40	1.3	.3	15.5	—	.6	70	22	.8	2	196	250	.10	.05	.5	71
Orange juice																	
Raw																	
All commercial varieties	88.3	45	.7	.2	10.4	.1	.4	11	17	.2	1	200	200	.09	.03	.4	50
California																	
Navels (winter oranges)	87.2	48	1.0	.1	11.3	(.1)	.4	11	18	.2	1	194	200	.09	.03	.4	61
Valencias (summer oranges)	87.8	47	1.0	.3	10.5	(.1)	.4	11	19	.3	1	190	200	.09	.03	.4	49
Florida																	
All commercial varieties	88.8	43	.6	.2	10.0	(.1)	.4	10	16	.2	1	206	200	.09	.03	.4	45
Early and midseason oranges (Hamlin, Parson Brown, Pineapple)	89.6	40	.5	.2	9.3	(.1)	.4	10	15	.2	1	208	200	.09	.03	.4	51
Late season (Valencias)	88.3	45	.6	.2	10.5	(.1)	.4	10	18	.2	1	203	200	.09	.03	.4	37
Temple	88.0	54	(.5)	(.2)	12.9	(.1)	.4	(10)	17	.2	1	—	(200)	.09	.03	.4	50
Canned																	
Unsweetened	87.4	48	.8	.2	11.2	.1	.4	10	18	.4	1	199	200	.07	.02	.3	40
Sweetened	86.5	52	.7	.2	12.2	.1	.4	(10)	18	.4	1	(199)	200	.07	.02	.3	40
Canned concentrate, unsweetened																	
Undiluted	42.0	223	4.1	1.3	50.7	.5	1.9	51	86	1.3	5	942	960	.39	.12	1.7	229
Diluted with 5 parts water, by volume	88.2	46	.8	.3	10.3	.1	.4	10	18	.3	1	192	200	.08	.02	.3	47
Frozen concentrate, unsweetened																	
Undiluted	58.2	158	2.3	.2	38.0	.2	1.3	33	55	.4	2	657	710	.30	.05	1.2	158
Diluted with 3 parts water, by volume	88.1	45	.7	.1	10.7	Trace	.4	9	16	.1	1	186	200	.09	.01	.3	45

Grapefruit
Raw
Pulp
Pink, red, white

All varieties	88.4	41	.5	.1	10.6	.2	.4	16	16	.4	1	135	80	0.04	.02	.2	38
California and Arizona (Marsh Seedless)	87.5	44	.5	.1	11.5	.2	.4	32	20	.4	1	135	10	.04	.02	.2	40
Florida, all varieties	89.1	38	.5	.1	9.9	.2	.4	15	15	.4	1	135	80	.04	.02	.2	37
Texas, all varieties	87.7	43	.5	.1	11.3	.2	.4	15	15	.4	1	135		.04	.02	.2	38
Pink and red																	
Seeded (Foster Pink)	88.6	40	.5	.1	10.4	.2	.4	16	16	.4	1	135	440	.04	.02	.2	39
Seedless (including Pink Marsh, Redblush)	88.6	40	.5	.1	10.4	.2	.4	16	16	.4	1	135	440	.04	.02	.2	36
White																	
Seeded (Duncan, other varieties)	88.2	41	.5	.1	10.8	.2	.4	16	16	.4	1	135	10	.04	.02	.2	38
Seedless (Marsh Seedless)	88.9	39	.5	.1	10.1	.2	.4	16	16	.4	1	135	10	.04	.02	.2	37
Juice																	
Pink, red, and white																	
All varieties	90.0	39	.5	.1	9.2	Trace	.2	9	15	.2	1	162	80	.04	.02	.2	38
California and Arizona (Marsh Seedless)	89.0	42	.4	.1	10.2	Trace	.3	9	15	.2	1	162	10	.04	.02	.2	40
Florida, all varieties	90.4	37	.5	.1	8.8	Trace	.2	9	15	.2	1	162	80	.04	.02	.2	37
Texas, all varieties	89.2	42	.5	.1	10.0	Trace	.2	9	15	.2	1	162		.04	.02	.2	38
Pink and red																	
Seeded (Foster Pink)	90.0	38	.5	.1	9.1	Trace	.3	9	15	.2	1	162	440	.04	.02	.2	39
Seedless (including Pink Marsh, Redblush)	90.0	39	.4	.1	9.3	Trace	.2	9	15	.2	1	162	440	.04	.02	.2	36
White																	
Seeded (Duncan, other varieties)	89.6	40	.5	.1	9.5	Trace	.3	9	15	.2	1	162	10	.04	.02	.2	38
Seedless (Marsh Seedless)	90.2	38	.5	.1	9.0	Trace	.2	9	15	.2	1	162	10	.04	.02	.2	37
Canned																	
Segments, solids and liquid																	
Water pack, with or without artificial sweetener.	91.3	30	.6	.1	7.6	.2	.4	13	14	.3	4	144	10	.03	.02	.2	30
Sirup pack	81.1	70	.6	.1	17.8	.2	.4	13	14	.3	1	135	10	.03	.02	.2	30
Juice																	
Unsweetened	89.2	41	.5	.1	9.8	Trace	.4	8	14	.4	1	162	10	.03	.02	.2	34
Sweetened	86.2	53	.5	.1	12.8	Trace	.4	8	14	.4	1	162	10	.03	.02	.2	31
Frozen concentrated juice																	
Unsweetened Undiluted	62.	145	1.9	.4	34.6	.1	1.1	34	60	.4	4	604	30	.14	.06	.7	138
Diluted with 3 parts water, by volume	89.3	41	.5	.1	9.8	Trace	.3	10	17	.1	1	170	10	.04	.02	.2	39

TABLE 10—Continued

TABLE 10—Continued

Food and description	Water (%)	Food energy (cals.)	Protein (gm.)	Fat (gm.)	Carbohydrate Total (gm.)	Fiber (gm.)	Ash (gm.)	Calcium (mg.)	Phosphorus (mg.)	Iron (mg.)	Sodium (mg.)	Potassium (mg.)	Vitamin A value (I.U.)	Thiamin (mg.)	Riboflavin (mg.)	Niacin (mg.)	Ascorbic acid (mg.)
Sweetened																	
Undiluted	57.	165	1.6	.3	40.2	.1	.9	28	50	.3	3	508	20	.12	.05	.6	116
Diluted with 3 parts water, by volume	87.8	47	.4	.1	11.4	Trace	.3	8	14	.1	1	144	10	.03	.01	.2	33
Dehydrated juice (crystals)																	
Dry form	1.0	378	4.8	1.0	90.3	.4	2.9	87	155	1.0	10	1,572	80	.36	.16	1.7	350
Prepared with water (1 lb. yields approx. 1 gal.)	89.5	40	.5	.1	9.6	Trace	.3	9	16	.1	1	167	10	.04	.02	.2	37
Grapefruit juice and orange juice blended																	
Canned																	
Unsweetened	88.7	43	.6	.2	10.1	.1	.4	10	15	.3	1	184	100	.05	.02	.2	34
Sweetened	86.9	50	.5	.1	12.2	.1	.4	10	15	.3	1	184	100	.05	.02	.2	34
Frozen concentrate, unsweetened																	
Undiluted	59.1	157	2.1	.5	37.1	.1	1.2	29	47	.4	2	623	380	.23	.03	1.1	144
Diluted with 3 parts water, by volume	88.4	44	.6	.1	10.5	Trace	.4	8	13	.1	Trace	177	110	.06	.01	.3	41

SOURCE: Composition of Foods—Raw, Processed, Prepared, USDA Agricultural Handbook 8, Revised 1963.
Numbers in parentheses denote values imputed—usually from another form of the food or from a similar food. Dashes denote lack of reliable data for a constituent believed to be present in measurable amount. Calculated values, as those based on a recipe, are not in parentheses.

TABLE 11. Desirable Weights for Men and Women, Aged 25 and Over

(Weight in pounds according to frame in indoor clothing)[1]

Men				Women			
Height with shoes, 1" heels				Height with shoes, 2" heels			
Feet Inches	Small frame	Medium frame	Large frame	Feet Inches	Small frame	Medium frame	Large frame
5 2	112–120	118–129	126–141	4 10	92–98	96–107	104–119
5 3	115–123	121–133	129–144	4 11	94–101	98–110	106–122
5 4	118–126	124–136	132–148	5 0	96–104	101–113	109–125
5 5	121–129	127–139	135–152	5 1	99–107	104–116	112–128
5 6	124–133	130–143	138–156	5 2	102–110	107–119	115–131
5 7	128–137	134–147	142–161	5 3	105–113	110–122	118–134
5 8	132–141	138–152	147–166	5 4	108–116	113–126	121–138
5 9	136–145	142–156	151–170	5 5	111–119	116–130	125–142
5 10	140–150	146–160	155–174	5 6	114–123	120–135	129–146
5 11	144–154	150–165	159–179	5 7	118–127	124–139	133–150
6 0	148–158	154–170	164–184	5 8	122–131	128–143	137–154
6 1	152–162	158–175	168–189	5 9	126–135	132–147	141–158
6 2	156–167	162–180	173–194	5 10	130–140	136–151	145–163
6 3	160–171	167–185	178–199	5 11	134–144	140–155	149–168
6 4	164–175	172–190	182–204	6 0	138–148	144–159	153–173

Source: Prepared by Metropolitan Life Insurance Company, 1960. Derived primarily from data of the Build and Blood Pressure Study, 1959.
1. For nude weight, deduct 5 to 7 pounds (male) and 2 to 4 pounds (female).

Energy Requirements and Physiological Strain

Energy expenditure during physical activity is estimated by direct calorimetry measurements of body heat production or by indirect estimations from oxygen consumption, heart rate, or pulmonary ventilation. The indirect measurements are then transformed to kilocalories of energy expenditures by utilizing standard caloric equivalents for oxygen consumed. Measurements obtained in this manner were used to establish relative energy requirements (see Table 12). (Harold B. Falls, Ph.D., Southwest Missouri State College, Springfield, "The relative energy requirements of various physical activities in relation to physiological strain." J. S. C. Med. Ass. 65, suppl. 1: 8–11, 1969. For reprint: Dr. Falls, Box 49, Southwest Missouri State College, Springfield, Missouri 65802.)

TABLE 12. Kilocalorie Energy Expenditure
per Minute for Typical
Sporting Activities

Activity	Energy expenditure (kcal. per min.)
Canoeing (2.5 mph)	3.0
Volleyball	3.5
Baseball	4.5
Ping-pong	4.6
Calisthenics	4.7
Golf	5.0
Archery	5.0
Dancing (rhumba)	7.0
Tennis	7.1
Horseback riding (trot)	8.0
Horseback riding (gallop)	10.0
Mountain climbing	10.0
Swim (breast stroke, 45 yd. / min.)	10.0
Squash	10.2
Cross-country running	10.6
Swim (backstroke, 45 yd. / min.)	11.0
Handball	11.0
Cycling (13 mph)	11.1
Swim, crawl (55 yd. / min.)	14.0
Skiing, level	15.9
Sprinting	23.0

Source: Adapted from Passmore and Durnin (170).

TABLE 13. Approximate Chemical Composition
of Orange Juice

Class of constituents	Constituents (number)	Total soluble solids (%)
Carbohydrates	7	76.0
Organic acids	7	9.6
Amino acids, free	17	5.4
Inorganic ions	14	3.2
Vitamins	14	2.5
Lipid constituents	18	1.2
Nitrogen bases and glutathione	5	.9
Flavonoids	1	.8
Volatile constituents	33	.38
Carotenoids	22	.013
Enzymes	12	
Total	150	100[1]

1. Approximate.

Daily Food and Nutrition Allowance

This diet plan is aimed at weight reduction and weight control while assuring reasonable nutritional adequacy. It does not prescribe a "set" menu. Rather it identifies a *daily* food allowance which may be divided and utilized according to individual selection and diet plans. This diet is relatively low in fat and cholesterol and should result in a reduction of plasma cholesterol as well as weight reduction with nutritional balance. It is desirable to eat breakfast daily. Avoid snacking. If you must snack, make it orange or grapefruit sections, or a carrot or celery stick. Weigh yourself and record weight daily; morning and night, under the same conditions.

12 oz. of citrus juice of your choice.

2 servings of fruit (i.e., 1 medium apple, 1 banana, 1 orange—your choice of 2).

8 oz. skim milk.

2 oz. dry cereal (not sugar-coated), use some of skim milk allowance and sweeten with artificial sweetener.

3 slices bread.

3 pats or equivalent of soft margarine.

Up to 2 oz. vegetable oil for cooking.

8 oz. lean meat, fish, or poultry or substitute 2 oz. cottage cheese for an equal meat portion. (Use fish and / or poultry four times per week. Broil meats or sauté in Teflon pan using small amounts of cooking oil. Avoid hot dogs and luncheon meats. Trim excess fat from meats.)

2 servings of your choice of vegetables (3/4 cup per serving).

Dessert (1 per day)—3/4 cup Jello plain, 1/2 cup ice milk, or a fruit choice.

Salad (for lunch or dinner)—1/4 wedge head of lettuce, 1 stalk (piece) of celery, 1 carrot (medium), 1 slice onion if desired. Use *low-cal* dressing only, of your choice.

Beverages (as desired)—artificial sweeteners as desired, "no-cal" drinks, skim milk with coffee or tea as desired. *Caution*: alcoholic beverages are not recommended. Their cost to you will be 1 mile of rapid walking for each 100 calories of alcohol consumed (i.e., 1 oz. of 100 proof bourbon equals 100 calories equals 1 mile walk at 4 miles per hour).

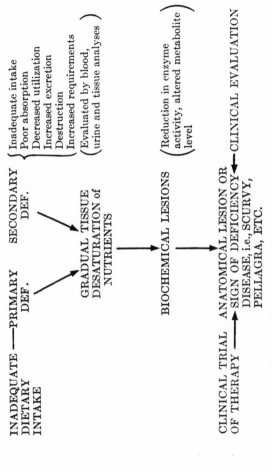

FIGURE 1. Clinical malnutrition—its development and evaluation. (Source: Krehl, 12.)

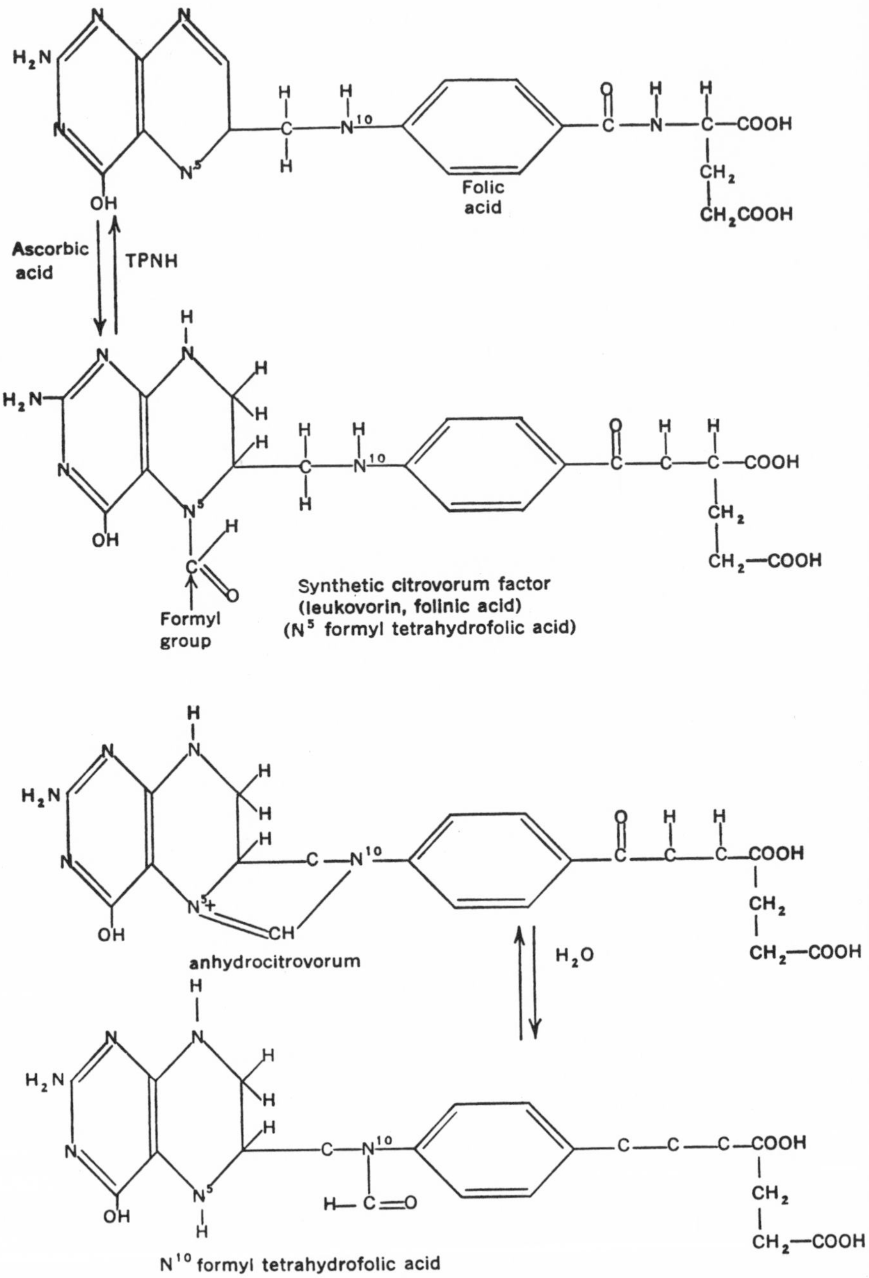

FIGURE 2. Structural formulas of folic acid, folinic acid, and some of the tetrahydrofolic acid coenzymes.

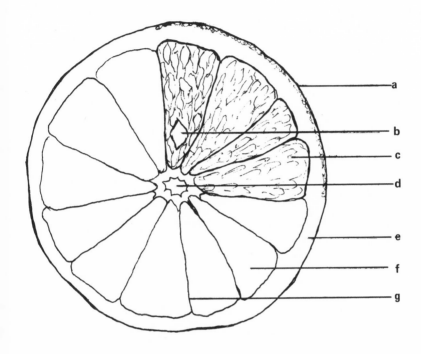

FIGURE 3 — SCHEMATIC VIEW OF THE CROSS SECTION OF AN ORANGE:

- a. Oil Sacs in flavedo
- b. Seed
- c. Juice Sacs
- d. Center Core
- e. Albedo
- f. Segment
- g. Segment membrane

Glossary

BRIX: Expressed in degrees, refers to the percentage by weight of soluble solids in the product. A measure for sugar.

BRIX / ACID RATIO: Direct ratio of Brix to amount of citric acid. An important indicator of flavor.

COLD PEEL: Sectionized fruit having peel removed by hand without any other treatment.

CONCENTRATE: Juice from which a substantial part of the moisture has been removed.

CUT OUT BRIX: In citrus section or salad packs, the combination of total natural sweetness from fruit plus the sugar added to it.

FREE AND SUSPENDED PULP: Pulp particles that are easily suspended upon shaking the container.

GLASS PACK: Container for pasteurized, single strength juice which precludes the growth of mold or yeast.

HERMETICALLY SEALED: Positive physical seal which does not allow oxygen to pass in or out.

HOT PEEL: Sectionized fruit having peel softened by heat before peeling.

PASTEURIZED: So treated by heat as to reduce organisms and inactivate enzymes.

PEEL OIL LEVEL: An expression of oil content in percentage of total product.

PH: A measure of hydrogen ion concentration (degree of acidity).

RAW JUICE: Juice extracted from fruit which has undergone no treatment or physical change.

RECONSTITUTED: Water added to product to approximately same level as moisture extracted in concentration process.

SINGLE STRENGTH ORANGE JUICE: Juice which has received no treatment relevant to concentration.

SYRUP FORMULATION: For chilled sections or salad, a combination of water, corn syrup, sugar, citric acid, and sodium benzoate.

References

1. *Citrus Fruits in Health and Disease*. The Florida Citrus Commission, Lakeland, Fla., 1948.
2. *Citrus Fruits in Health and Disease*. (Second Edition.) The Florida Citrus Commission, Lakeland, Fla., 1956.
3. Krehl, W. A.: "A Concept of Optimal Nutrition." Amer. J. Clin. Nutr. 4:646, 1956.
4. Cheraskin, E. and Ringsdorf, W. M., Jr.: "Predictive Medicine. 9. Diet." J. Amer. Geriat. Soc. 19:962, 1971.
5. Cheraskin, E. and Ringsdorf, W. M., Jr.: "Predictive Medicine. 3. An Ecologic Approach." J. Amer. Geriat. Soc. 19:505, 1971.
6. Cheraskin, E. and Ringsdorf, W. M., Jr.: "Predictive Medicine. 15. Epilogue." J. Amer. Geriat. Soc. 20:279, 1972.
7. Cheraskin, E. and Ringsdorf, W. M., Jr.: "Predictive Medicine. 14. Results." J. Amer. Geriat. Soc. 20:184, 1972.
8. Krehl, W. A.: "Nutritional Significance of Dietary Imbalance." Fed. Proc. 23:1059, 1964.
9. Pauling, L.: *Vitamin C and the Common Cold*. W. H. Freeman, San Francisco, 1970.
10. *Ten-State Nutrition Survey 1968–70*. U.S. Dept. of HEW, Hlth. Ser. & Men. Hlth. Adm., Center for Disease Control, Atlanta, Georgia 30333. (DPHEW Publication HMS 72-8134.)
11. Krehl, W. A.: "Contributions of Nutrition to Medicine and Health: Past and Potential." Amer. J. Clin. Nutr. 16:517, 1965.
12. Krehl, W. A.: "The Evaluation of Nutritional Status." Med. Clin. of North Amer. 48:1129, 1964.
13. Pearson, W. N.: "Biochemical Appraisal of Nutritional Status in Man." Amer. J. Clin. Nutr. 11:462, 1962.
14. Krehl, W. A. and Hodges, R. E.: "The Interpretation of Nutrition Survey Data." Amer. J. Clin. Nutr. 17:191, 1965.
15. *A Study of the Military Applicability of Research on Ascorbic Acid*. Life Sci. Res. Office, Red. Am. Soc. Exptl. Biol., Washington, D.C., 1963.
16. Browe, J. J.: "Provisions of Suitable and Sufficient Nutrition." In *Preventive Medicine* by Hilleboe, H. E. and Larimore, G. W., W. B. Saunders Co., Philadelphia, pp. 278–93, 1965.

17. *Dietary Levels of Households in the United States—Spring 1965 (A Preliminary Report.)* Agr. Res. Ser., ARS 62–17, U.S. Dept. Agr., 1968.

18. Briggs, G. M.: "Nutrition Education and Food Labels." Food and Nutrition News 44:April, 1973.

19. Recommended Dietary Allowances, Eighth Revised Edition, Food and Nutrition Board, National Research Council, National Academy of Sciences, Washington, D.C., 1974.

20. Harper, A. E.: "Carbohydrates in Human Nutrition." In *Symposium on Foods: Carbohydrates and Their Roles.* H. W. Schultz (Editor). AVI Publishing Co., Westport, Conn., 1969.

21. *Hunger, U.S.A. 1968.* A report by the Citizens' Board of Inquiry into Hunger and Malnutrition in the United States. New Community Press, Washington, D.C., 1968.

22. Davis, T. R. A., Gershoff, S. N., and Gamble, D. F.: "Review of Studies of Vitamin and Mineral Nutrition in the United States (1950–1968)." J. Nutr. Educ. 1:141, 1969.

23. Kelsay, J. L.: "A Compendium of Nutritional Status Studies and Dietary Evaluation Studies Conducted in the United States, 1957–1967." J. Nutr. 99:123, 1969.

24. Campbell, J. A.: "The Nutrition Survey of Canada." Canada J. Publ. Hlth. 61:156, 1970.

25. Williams, R. J.: *You Are Extraordinary.* Random House, N.Y., 1967.

26. Williams, R. J. and Deason, G.: "Individuality in Vitamin C Needs." Proc. Natl. Acad. Sci. U.S. 57:1638, 1967.

27. Smith, F. A., Trivas, G., Zuehlke, D. A., Lowinger, P., and Nghiem, T. L.: "Health Information during a Week of Television." New Engl. J. Med. 286:516, 1972.

28. McCord, C. P.: "Scurvy as an Occupational Disease (A Series)." J. Occup. Med.
    1. Introduction. J. Occup. Med. 13:1971.
    2. Early Sea Exploration. J. Occup. Med. 13:348, 1971.
    3. Scurvy during the Early Global Circum-navigations. J. Occup. Med. 13:393, 1971.
    4. Scurvy and the Nation's Men-of-War. J. Occup. Med. 13:441, 1971.
    5. Scurvy and the Merchant Marines. J. Occup. Med. 13:484, 1971.
    6. Scurvy Among the Whalers. J. Occup. Med. 13:543, 1971.
    7. Scurvy and the World's Armies. J. Occup. Med. 13:586, 1971.
    8. Scurvy and the Slave Trade. J. Occup. Med. 14:45, 1972.
    9. Scurvy in Polar Expeditions. J. Occup. Med. 14:232, 1972.
    10. Scurvy among Early American Western Migrants. J. Occup. Med. 14:321, 1972.
    11. Scurvy and Gold in Alaska. J. Occup. Med. 14:397, 1972.
    12. Scurvy in the Early American Colonies. J. Occup. Med. 14:556, 1972.

29. Stevenson, E. H.: "Importance of Vitamin C in the Diet." Report of Council on Foods and Nutrition. J.A.M.A. 160:1470, 1956.

30. Atkins, G. L., Dean, B. M., Griffin, W. J., and Watts, R. W. E.: "Quantitative Aspects of Ascorbic Acid Metabolism in Man." J. Biol. Chem. 239:2975, 1964.

31. Peterkofsky, B. and Undenfriend, S.: "Enzymatic Hydroxylation of Proline in Microsomal Polypeptide Leading to Formation of Collagen." Proc. Natl. Acad. Sci. 53:335, 1965.

32. Baker, E. M., Saari, J. C., and Tolbert, B. M.: "Ascorbic Acid Metabolism in Man." Amer. J. Clin. Nutr. 19:371, 1966.

33. Baker, E., Hodges, R. E., Hood, J., Sauberlich, H. E., and Marca, S. C.: "Metabolism of Ascorbic-1-14C Acid in Experimental Human Scurvy." Amer. J. Clin. Nutr. 22:549, 1969.

34. Baker, E. M., Sauberlich, H. E., Amos, W. H., and Tillotson, J. A.: "Use of Carbon-14 Labeled in Vitamins in Human Nutrition Studies: Pyridoxine and L-ascorbic Acid." J. Clin. Nutr. 18:302, 1966.
35. Tolbert, B. M., Chen, A. W., Bell, E. M., and Baker, E. M.: "Metabolism of L-Ascorbic-4-H Acid in Man." Amer. J. Clin. Nutr. 40:250, 1967.
36. Baker, E. M., Levandoski, N. G., and Sauberlich, H. E.: "Respiratory Catabolism in Man of the Degradative Intermediates of L-Ascorbic-1-C 14 Acid. (28371)." Proc. Soc. Exptl. Biol. Med. 109:737, 1962.
37. Lopez, A., Krehl, W. A., and Good, E.: "Influence of Time and Temperature on Ascorbic Acid Stability." J. Amer. Diet. Assoc. 50:308, 1967.
38. Bissett, O. W. and Berry, R. E.: "Ascorbic Acid Retention in Orange Juice as Related to Container Type." J. Food Sci. 40:178, 1975.
39. Huggart, R. L., Harman, D. A., and Moore, E. L.: "Ascorbic Acid Retention in Frozen Concentrated Citrus Juices." J. Amer. Diet. Assoc. 30:682, 1954.
40. Krehl, W. A. and Winters, R. W.: "Effect of Cooking Methods on Retention of Vitamins and Minerals in Vegetables." J. Amer. Diet. Assoc. 26:966, 1950.
41. Fincke, M. L., McGregor, M. A., Storvick, C. A., and Woods, E.: "Ascorbic Acid Content of Foods as Served." J. Amer. Diet. Assoc. 24:957, 1948.
42. Vilter, R. W.: "Folic Acid." In *Modern Nutrition in Health and Disease* by Wohl, M. D. and Goodhart, R. S., Lea and Febiger, Philadelphia, Pa., pp. 273–85, 1968.
43. Luhby, A. L. and Cooperman, J. M.: "Folic Acid Deficiency in Man and Its Interrelationships with Vitamin B-12 Metabolism." Adv. Metab. Disord. 1:263, 1964.
44. Herbert, V. (with the technical assistance of R. Fisher and B. J. Koontz): "The Assay and Nature of Folic Acid Activity in Human Serum." J. Clin. Invest. 40:81, 1961.
45. Temperley, I. J. and Horner, N.: "Effect of Ascorbic Acid on the Serum Folic Acid Estimation." J. Clin. Path. 19:43, 1966.
46. Herbert, V.: "Studies of Folate Deficiency in Man." Proc. Roy. Soc. Med. 57:379, 1964.
47. Herbert, V.: "Biochemical and Hematologic Lesions in Folic Acid Deficiency." Amer. J. Clin. Nutr. 20:562, 1967.
48. Butterworth, C. E., Baugh, C. M., and Krumdieck, C.: "A Study of Folate Absorption and Metabolism in Man Utilizing Carbon-14 Labeled Polyglutamates Synthesized by the Solid Phase Method." J. Clin. Invest. 48:1131, 1969.
49. Grossoweiz, N., Rachmilewitz, M., and Izak, G.: "Absorption of Pteroylglutamate and Dietary Folates in Man." Amer. J. Clin. Nutr. 25:1135, 1972.
50. Perry, J. and Chanarin, I.: "Absorption and Utilization of Polyglutamyl Forms of Folate in Man." Brit. Med. J. 4:546, 1968.
51. Perry, J. and Chanarin, I.: "Intestinal Absorption of Reduced Folate Compounds in Man." Brit. J. Haematol. 18:329, 1970.
52. Herbert, V.: "Minimal Daily Adult Folate Requirement." AMA Arch. Int. Med. 110:649, 1962.
53. Baker, H., Frank, O., Feingold, S., Ziffer, H., Gellene, R. A., Leevy, C. M., and Sobotka, H.: "The Fate of Orally and Parenterally Administered Folates." Amer. J. Clin. Nutr. 17:88, 1965.
54. Rosenbert, I. H. and Godwin, H. A.: "The Digestion and Absorption of Dietary Folate." Gastroenterology 60:445, 1971.
55. Santini, R., Brewster, C., and Butterworth, C. E., Jr.: "The Distribution of Folic Acid Active Compounds in Individual Foods." Amer. J. Clin. Nutr. 14:305, 1964.
56. Hoppner, K., Lampi, B., and Perrin, D. E.: "The Free and Total Folate Activity in Foods Available on the Canadian Market." J. Inst. Can. Sci. Tech. Aliment. 5:60, 1972.

57. Dong, F. M. and Oace, S. M.: "Folate Distribution in Fruit Juices." J. Amer. Diet. Assoc. 62:162, 1973.

58. Nelson, E. W., DeFord, J., Streiff, R. R., and Cerda, J. J.: "Studies of Comparative Bioavailability of Water Soluble Vitamins: A New Method." Western Hemisphere Nutrition Congress (Abstracts), Miami Beach, Fla., p. 42, 1974.

59. Streiff, R. R.: "Folate Levels in Citrus and Other Juices." J. Amer. Clin. Nutr. 24:1390–98, 1971.

60. Butterworth, E. E., Jr., Santini, R., Jr., and Fronmeyer, W. B., Jr.: "The Pteroyl-glutamate Components of American Diets as Determined by Chromatographic Fractionation." J. Clin. Invest. 42:1929, 1963.

61. Reynolds, E. H.: "Anticonvulsants, Folic Acid, and Epilepsy." The Lancet, pp. 1376–78, June 16, 1973.

62. Haghshanass, M. and Dodd, B. R.: "Serum Folate Levels during Anticonvulsant Therapy with Dephenylhydantoin." J. Amer. Geriat. Soc. 21:275–77, 1973.

63. Balaghi, M. and Pearson, W. N.: "Alterations in the Metabolism of 2-14C-Thiazole-Labeled Thiamine by the Rat Induced by a High Fat Diet or Thyroxine." J. Nutr. 90:161, 1966.

64. Williams, R. D., Mason, H. L., Smith, B. F., and Wilder, R. M.: "Induced Thiamine (Vitamin B₁) Deficiency and Thiamine Requirement of Man: Further Observations." AMA Arch. Int. Med. 69:721, 1942.

65. Food and Agriculture Organization / World Health Organization of the United Nations: "Requirements of Vitamin A, Thiamine, Riboflavin, and Niacin." FAO Nutr. Meet. Rep. Ser. No. 41; WHO Tech. Rep. Ser. No. 362, p. 32, Rome, 1967.

66. Leaf, A. and Santos, R. F.: "Physiologic Mechanisms in Potassium Deficiency." New Engl. J. Med. 264:335, 1961.

67. Kosman, M. E.: "Management of Potassium Problems during Long Term Diuretic Therapy." J.A.M.A. 230:743–48, 1974.

68. Alper, C.: "Fluid and Electrolyte Balance." In *Modern Nutrition in Health and Disease* by Wohl, M. D. and Goodhart, R. S., Lea and Febiger, Philadelphia, Pa., pp. 404–25, 1968.

69. Galbraith, J. M.: "Bendroflumethiazide in Hypertension and Edematous States (Use in Office Practice)." N.Y. State J. Med. 62:1209, 1962.

70. Bare, W. W. and Baird, H. L.: "Hypertension and Edema in the Aged: Observations on the Use of a Meprobamate-Hydrochlorthiazide Concentration." J. Amer. Geriat. Soc. 9:968, 1961.

71. Bruner, R. C. and Palmer, G. H.: "Citrus Bioflavonoids in Health and Disease." Review with references B-702, B-703, B-724, B-761, and B-768. Sunkist Growers, Ontario, Calif., p. 12, 1961.

72. Vilter, R. W.: "Vitamin C (Ascorbic Acid) and Bioflavonoids." In *Modern Nutrition in Health and Disease* by Wohl, M. D. and Goodhart, R. S., Lea and Febiger, Philadelphia, Pa., pp. 296–304, 1968.

73. Robbins, R. C.: "Effect of Vitamin C and Flavonoids on Blood Cell Aggregation and Capillary Resistance." Intern. Z. Vitaminforsch. 36:10, 1966.

74. American Academy of Pediatrics Committee on Nutrition: "Infantile Scurvy and Nutritional Rickets in the United States." Pediatrics 29:646, 1962.

75. Ossofsky, H. J.: "Infantile Scurvy." Amer. J. Dis. Child. 109:173, 1965.

76. Woodruff, C.: "The Increasing Incidence of Scurvy in the Nashville Area." Report to Council on Foods and Nutrition, J.A.M.A. 161:448, 1956.

77. Follis, R. H., Jr.: *The Pathology of Nutritional Disease*. Charles C. Thomas Publ., Springfield, Ill., 1948.

78. Gutelius, M. F.: "The Problem of Iron Deficiency Anemia in Preschool Negro Children." Publ. Hlth. Rep. 8:213, 1968.

79. Filer, L. J. and Martinez, G. A.: "Caloric and Iron Intake by Infants in the United States. An Evaluation of 4,000 Representative Six-Month-Olds." Clin. Pediat. 3:633, 1963.

80. Gorton, M. K. and Bradley, J. E.: "The Treatment of Nutritional Anemia in Infancy and Childhood with Oral Iron and Ascorbic Acid." J. Pediatrics 45:1, 1954.

81. Conrad, M. E. and Schade, S. G.: "Ascorbic Acid in Iron Absorption: A Role for Hydrochloric Acid and Bile." Gastroenterology 55:25, 1968.

82. Whelen, W. S., Fraser, D., Robertson, E. C., and Tomczak, H.: "The Rising Incidence of Scurvy in Infants—A Challenge to the Physician and the Community." Canada Med. J. 78:177, 1958.

83. Schweigart, H. A.: "Why is Natural Vitamin C Superior to Synthetic Vitamin C?" Hippokrates 26:151, 1955.

84. Prokop, L.: "The Effect of Natural Vitamin C on Oxygen Utilization and Circulatory Economy." Neue Zeitschr. Arztl. Fortbild. pp. 448–55, 1960.

85. Ratner, B., Untracht, S., Malone, J., and Restina, M.: "Allergenicity of Modified and Processed Foodstuffs. 4. Orange: Allergenicity of Oranges Studied in Man." J. Pediatrics 43:421, 1953.

86. Joslin, C. L. and Bradley, J. E.: "Studies on Orange Juice, Orange Juice Concentrate and Orange Peel Oil in Infants and Children." J. Pediatrics 39:325, 1951.

87. Lawrence, R. A. and Hawley, E. E.: "A Comparative Study of the Acceptance and Tolerance of Orange Juice and 'Commercial Instant Breakfast Drink' by 114 Infants." Amer. J. Clin. Nutr. 10:137, 1962.

88. Mott, G. A., Ross, R. H., and Smith, D. J.: "A Study of Vitamin C and D Intake of Infants in the Metropolitan Vancouver Area." Canada J. Publ. Hlth. 55:341, 1964.

89. Hodges, R. E. and Krehl, W. A.: "Nutritional Status of Teenagers in Iowa." Amer. J. Clin. Nutr. 17:200, 1965.

90. O'Sullivan, D. J., Callaghan, N., Ferris, J. B., Finucane, J. F., and Hagerty, M.: "Ascorbic Acid Deficiency in the Elderly." Irish J. Med. Sci., 7th ser., 1:151, 1968.

91. Andrews, J., Letcher, M., and Brook, M.: "Vitamin C Supplementation in the Elderly: A 17-Month Trial in an Old Persons' Home." Brit. Med. J. 2:416, 1969.

92. Allen, R. J. L. and Brook, M.: "The Variability of Vitamin C in Our Diet." Brit. J. Nutr. 22:555, 1968.

93. Avioli, L. V., McDonald, J. E., and Lee, S. W.: "The Influence of Age in the Intestinal Absorption of 47 Ca in Woman and Its Relation to 45 Ca Absorption in Postmenopausal Osteoporosis." J. Clin. Invest. 44:1960, 1965.

94. Heaney, R. P.: "A Unified Concept of Osteoporosis." Amer. J. Med. 39:877, 1965.

95. Leitch, I. and Aitkin, F. C.: "The Estimation of Calcium Requirement: A Re-examination." Nutr. Abstr. Rev. 29:393, 1959.

96. Cohen, M. M. and Duncan, A. M.: "Ascorbic Acid Nutrition in Gastroduodenal Disorders." Brit. Med. J. 5578:516, 1967.

97. Hansky, J. and Allmand, F.: "Gastro-intestinal Bleeding. The Role of Vitamin C." Austral. Ann. Med. 18:248, 1969.

98. Council on Foods and Nutrition: "Diet and Coronary Heart Disease." J.A.M.A. 222:1647, 1972.

99. *1973 Heart Facts.* The American Heart Association. 44 East 23 St., New York, N.Y.

100. Kannel, W. B., Dawber, T. R., Kagan, A., Revotskie, N., and Stokes, J.: "Factors of Risk in the Development of Coronary Artery Disease: 6-Year Follow-Up Experience." Ann. Intern. Med. 55:33, 1961.

101. Connor, W. E., Hodges, R. E., and Bleiler, R. E.: "Effect of Dietary Cholesterol upon Serum Lipids in Man." J. Lab. Clin. Med. 57:331, 1961.
102. Page, I. H. and Stamler, J.: "Diet and Coronary Heart Disease (1)." Mod. Conc. Cardiov. Dis. 37:119, 1968.
103. Page, I. H. and Stamler, J.: "Diet and Coronary Heart Disease (11)." Mod. Conc. Cardiov. Dis. 37:125, 1968.
104. Strong, J. P., Eggen, D. A., Oalmann, M. D., Richards, M. L., and Tracy, R. E.: "Pathology and Epidemiology of Atherosclerosis." J. Amer. Diet. Assoc. 62:262, 1973.
105. Taylor, H. L., Klepetar, E., Keys, A., Parlin, W., Blackburn, H., and Punchner, J.: "Death Rates among Physically Active and Sedentary Employees of the Railroad Industry." Amer. J. Publ. Hlth. 52:1697, 1962.
106. Jenkins, C. D.: "Psychologic and Social Precursors of Coronary Disease." (First of Two Parts) New Engl. J. Med. 284:244, 1971.
107. Jenkins, C. D.: "Psychologic and Social Precursors of Coronary Disease." (Second of Two Parts) New Engl. J. Med. 284:307, 1971.
108. Keys, A., Grande, F., and Anderson, J. T.: "Fiber and Pectin in the Diet and Serum Cholesterol Concentration in Man." Proc. Soc. Exptl. Biol. Med. 106:555, 1961.
109. Wells, A. F. and Ershoff, B. H.: "Beneficial Effects of Pectin in Prevention of Hypercholesterolemia and Increase in Liver Cholesterol in Cholesterol-Fed Rats." J. Nutr. 74:87, 1961.
110. Wells, A. F. and Ershoff, B. H.: "Protective Effect of Pectin Against the Increase in Liver and Plasma Cholesterol Induced by Cholesterol Feeding in the Immature Male Rat." Fed. Proc. 18:2171, 1959.
111. Spittle, C. R.: "Atherosclerosis and Vitamin C." The Lancet, p. 1280, Dec. 11, 1971.
112. Spittle, C. R.: "Atherosclerosis and Vitamin C." The Lancet, p. 798, April 8, 1972.
113. Sokoloff, B., Hor, M., Saelhof, C. C., Wrxolek, T., and Imai, T.: "Aging, Atherosclerosis and Ascorbic Acid Metabolism." J. Amer. Geriat. Soc. 14:1239, 1966.
114. Sokoloff, B., Hor, M., Saelhof, C., McConnell, B., and Imai, T.: "Effect of Ascorbic Acid on Certain Blood Fat Metabolism Factors in Animals and Man." J. Nutr. 91:107, 1967.
115. Pelletier, O.: "Smoking and Vitamin C Levels in Humans." Amer. J. Clin. Nutr. 21:1259, 1968.
116. Brook, M. and Grimshaw, J. J.: "Vitamin Concentration of Plasma and Leukocytes as Related to Smoking Habit, Age, and Sex of Humans." Amer. J. Clin. Nutr. 21:1254, 1968.
117. Bailey, D. A., Carron, A. V., Teece, R. G., and Wehner, H. J.: "Vitamin C Supplementation Related to Physiological Response to Exercise in Smoking and Non-smoking Subjects." Amer. J. Clin. Nutr. 23:905, 1970.
118. Ginter, E.: "Cholesterol: Vitamin C Controls Its Transformation to Bile Acids." Science 179:702, 1973.
119. Ginter, E.: "Atherosclerosis and Vitamin C." The Lancet, p. 1233, June 3, 1972.
120. Ginter, E., Babala, J., and Cerven, J.: "Effect of Chronic Hypovitaminosis C on the Metabolism of Cholesterol and Atherogenesis in Guinea Pigs." J. Atheroscler. Res. 10:341, 1969.
121. Ginter, E., Ondreicka, R., Bobek, P., and Simko, V.: "Influence of Chronic Vitamin C Deficiency on Fatty Acid Composition of Blood Serum, Liver Triglycerides and Cholesterol Esters in Guinea Pigs." J. Nutr. 99:261, 1969.

122. Coffee Drinking and Acute Myocardial Infarction: Report from the Boston Collaborative Drug Surveillance Program, Lancet 2, 1278–81, 1972.

123. Ischaemic Heart Disease Registers: Report of the 5th Working Group, Copenhagen, World Health Organization, April 26–29, 1971.

124. Paul, O.: "Coffee Drinking and Myocardial Infarction." Postgrad. Med. 44:196, 1968.

125. Coffee and Myocardial Infarction: A Report from the Boston Collaborative Drug Surveillance Program, Boston University Medical Center. New Engl. J. Med. 289:63–67, 1973.

126. Mayer, J.: "Some Aspects of the Problem of Regulation of Food Intake and Obesity." New Engl. J. Med. 274:610, 1966.

127. Van Itallie, T. B. and Campbell, R. C.: "Multidisciplinary Approach to the Problem of Obesity." J. Amer. Diet. Assoc. 61:385, 1972.

128. Van Itallie, T. B. and Hashim, S. A.: "Obesity in an Age of Caloric Anxiety." Mod. Med. pp. 89–96, Nov. 30, 1970.

129. Lawrence, A. M.: "Obesity—New Happenings." Food and Nutrition News 43:8–9, May–June, 1972.

130. Seltzer, C. C. and Mayer, J.: "A Simple Criterion of Obesity." Postgrad. Med. 38:A101, 1965.

131. Walker, H. C., Jr.: "Obesity: Its Complications and Sequalae." Arch. Int. Med. 93:951, 1954.

132. Abraham, S. and Nordsieck, M.: "Relationship of Excess Weight in Children and Adults." Publ. Health Rep. 75:263, 1960.

133. Johnson, M. L., Burke, B. S., and Mayer, J.: "Relative Importance of Inactivity and Overeating in Energy Balance of Obese High School Girls." Amer. J. Clin. Nutr. 4:37, 1956.

134. Bullen, B. A., Reed, R. B., and Mayer, J.: "Physical Activity of Obese and Adolescent Girls Appraised by Motion Picture Sampling." Amer. J. Clin. Nutr. 14:211, 1964.

135. Moore, M. E., Stunkard, A., and Srole, L.: "Obesity, Social Class and Mental Illness." J.A.M.A. 181:962, 1962.

136. Seltzer, C. C. and Mayer, J.: "Body Build and Obesity—Who are the Obese?" J.A.M.A. 189:677, 1964.

137. Seltzer, C. C., Goldman, R. F., and Mayer, J.: "Triceps Skinfold as Predictive Measure of Body Density and Body Fat in Obese Adolescent Girls." Pediatrics 36:212, 1965.

138. Westerfeld, W. W. and Schulman, M. P.: "Metabolism and Caloric Value of Alcohol." J. Amer. Med. Assoc. 170:197, 1959.

139. Cooper, K. H.: "Guidelines in the Management of the Exercising Patient." J.A.M.A. 211: March 9, 1970.

140. Cureton, T. K.: "Diet Related to Athletics and Physical Fitness." Part 3. J. Phys. Ed. 57:6, 1959.

141. Consolazio, C. F.: "Nutritional Basis for Optimal Performance." U.S. Army Medical Research and Nutritional Laboratory. Paper presented at 9th National Conference on the Medical Aspects of Sports, November, 1967.

142. "Diet, Exercise, and Endurance." Nutr. Rev. 30:86, 1972.

143. Maternal Nutrition and the Course of Pregnancy, Summary Report, National Academy of Sciences, H.S. Department of Health, Education and Welfare. Rockville, Md., p. 5, 1970.

144. Hunter, C. A., Jr.: "Iron-Deficiency Anemia in Pregnancy." Surg. Gynecol. Obst. 110:210, 1960.

145. Javert, C. T.: "Decidual Bleeding in Pregnancy." Ann. N.Y. Acad. Sci. 61:700, 1955.

146. Murphy, H. S.: "The Treatment of Threatened Abortion." J. Med. Soc. New Jersey 58:60, 1961.
147. Quick, A. J.: "The Third Hemostatic Vitamin." Wisc. Med. J. 71:175, 1972.
148. Clemetson, C. A. B. and Blair, L. M.: "Capillary Strength of Women with Menorrhagia." Amer. J. Obst. Gynec. 83:1269, 1962.
149. Shils, M. E. and Goodhart, R. S.: "The Flavonoids in Biology and Medicine. (A Critical Review)." National Vitamin Foundation, Inc., N.Y., N.Y., January 1956.
150. Emerson, K., Jr., Saxena, B. N., and Poindexter, E. L.: "Caloric Cost of Normal Pregnancy." Obst. Gynec. 40:786, 1972.
151. Streiff, R. R. and Little, A. B.: "Folic Acid Deficiency in Pregnancy." New Engl. J. Med. 276:776, 1967.
152. Hibbard, B. M., Hibbard, E. D., and Jeffcoate, T. N. A.: "Folic Acid in Reproduction." Acta Obst. Gynec. Scand. 44:375, 1965.
153. Lawrence, C. and Klipstein, F. A.: "Megaloblastic Anemia of Pregnancy in New York City." Ann. Intern. Med. 66:25, 1967.
154. Alperin, J. B., Hutchinson, H. T., and Levin, W. C.: "Studies of Folic Acid Requirements in Megaloblastic Anemia of Pregnancy." AMA Arch. Int. Med. 117:681, 1966.
155. Giles, C.: "An Analysis of 335 Cases of Megaloblastic Anemia of Pregnancy and the Puerperium." J. Clin. Path. 19:1, 1966.
156. Kitay, D. Z., Hogan, W. J., Eberle, B., and Mynt, T.: "Neutrophil Hypersegmentation and Folic Acid Deficiency in Pregnancy." Amer. J. Obst. Gynec. 104:1163, 1969.
157. Chisholm, M. and Sharp, A. A.: "Formininoglutamic Acid Excretion in Anemia of Pregnancy." Brit. Med. J. 11:1366, 1964.
158. Ball, E. W. and Giles, C. J.: "Folic Acid and Vitamin B_{12} Levels in Pregnancy and Their Relation to Megaloblastic Anemia." J. Clin. Pathol. 17:165, 1964.
159. Edelstein, T., Stevens, K., Baumslag, N., and Metz, J.: "Effect of Supplementation on Tests of Folic Acid Deficiency in Pregnancy." J. Obst. Gynec. Brit. Cwlth. 75:133, 1968.
160. Streiff, R. R.: "Folate Deficiency and Oral Contraceptives." J.A.M.A. 214:105, 1970.
161. Cheraskin, E. and Ringsdorf, W. M., Jr.: "Predictive Medicine. 12. The Oral Cavity." J. Amer. Geriat. Soc. 20:88, 1972.
162. Shaw, J. H.: "Diet Regulations for Caries Prevention." Nutrition News. Vol. 36, No. 1, Feb. 1973.
163. Cheraskin, E. and Ringsdorf, W. M., Jr.: "Biology of the Orthodontic Patient. 3. Relationship of Chronologic and Dental Age in Terms of Vitamin C State." The Angle Orthodontist 42:56, 1972.
164. Ringsdorf, W. M. and Cheraskin, E.: "A Rapid and Simple Lingual Ascorbic Acid Test." G. P. 25:106, 1962.
165. Cheraskin, E. and Ringsdorf, W. M., Jr.: "A Lingual Vitamin C Test: 1. Reproducibility." Interntl. J. Vit. Res. 38:114, 1968.
166. Cheraskin, E. and Ringsdorf, W. M., Jr.: "A Lingual Vitamin C Test. 3. Relationship to Plasma Ascorbic Acid Level." Interntl. J. Vit. Res. 38:123, 1968.
167. McDonald, B. S.: "Gingivitis-Ascorbic Acid Deficiency in the Navajo. 3. Dietary Aspects." J. Amer. Diet. Assoc. 43:331, 1963.
168. Nizel, A. E.: "Diet in Oral Surgery." Oral Surg. 14:539, 1961.
169. Shannon, I. L. and Gibson, W. A.: "Blood and Urine Ascorbic Acid Levels in Subjects Classified as to Dental Caries Experience." Arch. Oral Biol. 9:371, 1964.
170. Passmore, B. and Durnin, J. V.: *Energy, Work and Leisure.* Heinemann Books, London, 1967.

171. Cheraskin, E. and Ringsdorf, W. M., Jr.: "What Does the Dental Family Eat? A Study of Refined Carbohydrate Consumption." J. Ala. Den. Assoc. 56:32, 1972.

172. Moore, C. V.: "The Importance of Nutritional Factors in the Pathogenesis of Iron-Deficiency Anemia." Amer. J. Clin. Nutr. 3:3, 1959.

173. Chingarina, L. A.: "The Level of Serum Iron in Preschool Children Depending Upon the Degree of Vitamin C Deficiency." Vop. Pitan. 26:81, 1967.

174. Majaj, A. S., Dinning, J. S., Axxam, S. A., and Darby, W. J.: "Vitamin E Responsive Megaloblastic Anemia in Infants with Protein-Calorie Malnutrition." Amer. J. Clin. Nutr. 12:374, 1963.

175. Vilter, R. W., Will, J. J., Wright, T., and Rullman, D.: "Interrelationships of Vitamin B_{12}, Folic Acid and Ascorbic Acid in Megaloblastic Anemia." Amer. J. Clin. Nutr. 12:130, 1963.

176. Vilter, R. W., Will, J. J., Wright, T., and Rullman, D.: "Interrelationships of Vitamin B_{12} in Methionine Biosynthesis in Avian Liver." J. Biol. Chem. 239:2545, 1964.

177. Cox, E. V., Meynell, M. J., Cook, W. T., and Gaddic, R.: "Scurvy and Anemia." Amer. J. Med. 32:240, 1962.

178. Horrigan, D. L. and Harris, J. W.: "Pyridoxine-Responsive Anemia: Analysis of 62 Cases." Adv. Int. Med. 12:103, 1964.

179. Kahn, S. B. and Brodsky, I.: "Metabolic Interrelationships Between Vitamin B_{12} and Ascorbic Acid in Pernicious Anemia." Blood 21:55, 1968.

180. Selye, H.: "On Just Being Sick." Nutrition Today 5:2, 1970.

181. Selye, H.: *In Vivo: The Case for Supramolecular Biology—No. 2.* Liveright Publ. Corp., N.Y., 1967.

182. Chalopin, H., Mouton, M., and Ratsimamanga, A. R.: "Some Interrelations Between Ascorbic Acid and Adreno-Cortical Function." Work Rev. Nutr. and Diet., Vol. 6, p. 165 (S. Karger, Basel / N.Y.), 1966.

183. Wolf, S.: "Emotions and the Autonomic Nervous System." Arch. Intern. Med. 126:1024, 1970.

184. Brock, J. F.: "Nature, Nurture, and Stress in Health and Disease." The Lancet, April 1972.

185. Baker, E. M.: "Vitamin C Requirements in Stress." Amer. J. Clin. Nutr. 20:583, 1967.

186. Van Huss, W. D.: "The Effects of Natural and Synthetic Vitamin C on Work Performance." East Lansing, Mich. State Univ., Human Energy Research Laboratory (N.D.).

187. Braun, I. G.: "Vitamin A: Excess, Deficiency, Requirement, Metabolism and Misuse." Pediat. Clin. N. Amer. 9:935, 1962.

188. Anderson, T. W., Reid, D. B. W., and Beaton, G. H.: "Vitamin C and the Common Cold: A Double-Blind Trial." Can. Med. Assoc. J. 107:503, 1972.

189. Beaton, G. H. and Whalen, S.: "Vitamin C and the Common Cold." Can. Med. Assoc. J. 105:335, 1971.

190. Wilson, C. W. M. and Loh, H. S.: "Common Cold and Vitamin C." The Lancet, p. 638, March 24, 1973.

191. Ritzel, G.: "Ascorbic Acid and Infections of the Respiratory Tract." Helv. Med. Acta 28:63, 1961.

192. Herjanic, M. and Moss-Herjanic, B. L.: "Ascorbic Acid Test in Psychiatric Patients." J. Schizophrenia 1:257, 1967.

193. Ting, S. V., Moore, E. L., McAllister, J. W., Streiff, R. R., Hsu, J. N. C., and Hill, E. C.: "Nutrient Assay of Florida Frozen Concentrated Orange Juice for Nutrition Labeling." Proc. Florida State Hort. Soc. 87:206–9, 1974.

194. Scala, J.: "Fiber—The Forgotten Nutrient." Food Technology 28(1):34–36, 1975.

References

195. Burkitt, D. P., Walker, A. R. P., and Painter, N. S.: "Dietary Fiber and Disease." J.A.M.A. 229(8):1068–74, 1974.
196. Eastwood, M. A.: "Medical and Dietary Management." Clinics in Gastroenterology 4(1):85–97, 1975.